The Drama of Fluorine
ARCH ENEMY OF MANKIND

I0113893

Abstract

Since the 1920s, modern science has known the dangers of fluoride poisoning. Sadly, this truth is continually hidden and ignored. Here is the effort of one man to benefit mankind.

By Leo Spira M.D., Ph.D. (Med.) 1953

This edition 2022 by Steve Fonseca

fonseca.steve@gmail.com

The Drama of Fluorine

ARCH ENEMY OF MANKIND

by

Leo Spira, M.D, Ph.D. (Med.)

Edition Notice:
- *Edition 2022 by Steve Fonseca USA*
- *This edition contains images of the cover and author's picture as originally published.*
- *The editor added an Addendum in this version.*
- *This edition was made in order to have a digitally searchable copy of this important work and to honor the author.*
- *May his dedication, hard work, and courage be always acknowledged.*

Originally Published 1953
by LEE FOUNDATION FOR NUTRITIONAL RESEARCH
Milwaukee 3, Wisconsin
Copyright 1953, by Dr. Leo Spira
Printed in the United States of America

Published 2022 by MollyPeterBooks
New York, USA

ISBN: 978-1-958689-00-4

The Drama Of Fluorine

ARCH ENEMY OF MANKIND

by

Leo Spira, M.D., Ph.D. (Med.)

1953

Published by

LEE FOUNDATION FOR NUTRITIONAL RESEARCH

Milwaukee 3, Wisconsin
Price - $2.00

Original Cover 1953

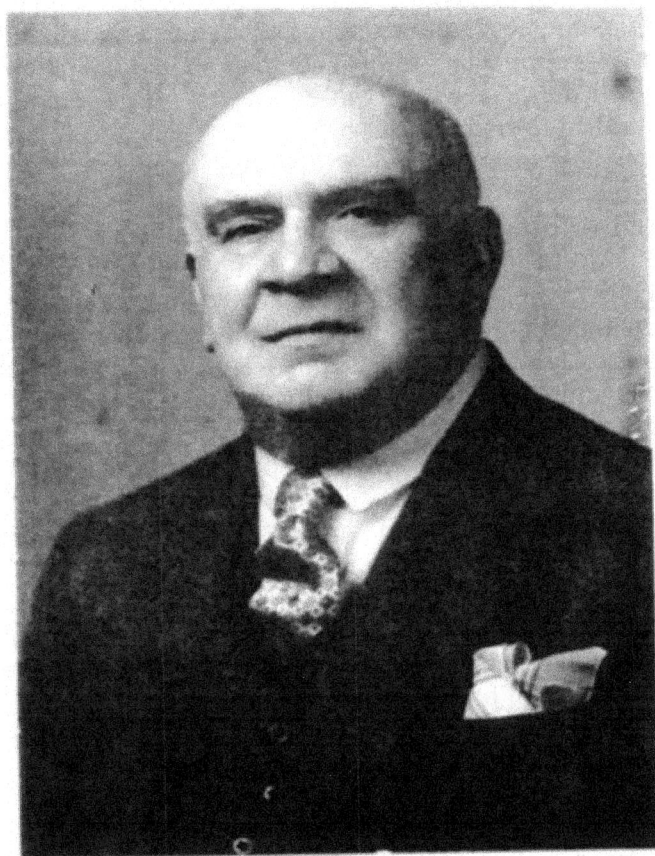

LEO SPIRA, M.D., Ph.D. (Med.)

PREFACE

The problem of fluorine is the subject of heated discussion all over the country at the present time, in the large city, the provincial town, and the remote village. An enlightened nation, brought up to use its own intelligence, refuses point blank to be told without adequate explanation what people should or should not do in matters affecting the health of each one of them. When it is proposed to tamper with their drinking-water by altering its chemical composition, they insist on being given facts based on unbiased studies carried out by competent investigators. In short, the nation wants to know whether any risk of injury to health is involved.

The information so far divulged about the problem of fluorine is, however, extremely biased. When conveyed through the remorseless exploitation of scanty knowledge, the facts have in many cases been grossly distorted. Incessantly repeated to unsuspecting listeners, they might in the absence of contradiction easily be accepted as the truth, the whole truth, and nothing but the truth.

There is, to be sure, plenty of opposition from individual groups organized for the purpose all over the country, but so far little help has been forthcoming from amongst those qualified to speak with some degree of authority on the hotly-disputed subject. All the more credit is due to those brave and upright men and women who in their lonely fight have spared no effort in an endeavor, often under most difficult conditions, to open the eyes of the nation. To them belongs the honour of having succeeded in keeping the question open until support would come in their gallant fight against the risk of the deteriorated health of future generations.

> "He that walketh righteously, and speaketh uprightly … Bread shall be given him; and his waters shall be sure."
>
> Isiah, Chapter 33, Verse 16

The purpose of this book is to help the general public to arrive at a better understanding than was hitherto possible of the issue involved in the controversy. "The Drama of Fluorine" is, in the main, a condensed summary of 34 papers which I published in various medical journals in this country, in Great Britain, and on the Continent of Europe. They were written for the medical profession and they have, I hope, caught the eye of some amongst them. There is, therefore, no need for me to apologize to my professional brethren for writing a book in a non-technical language on a problem which is sure to interest the general public as much as it should interest every medical man and dentist.

I wish to emphasize as strongly as I can that the information here supplied is authentic and based on facts which can easily be verified. Throughout the whole of my work, I insisted on having impartial witnesses, so to enable me to nip in the bud any unfriendly suggestion that it is based on "imagination and psychological effects".

In the course of my research on the subject of fluorine, I had to overcome many obstacles, but I was also fortunate in having the help of many people. Outstanding amongst them was Professor Samson Wright, Head of the Department of Physiology, Middlesex Hospital Medical School, London, England, who gave me the sorely needed chance of finding out whether the results of my previously recorded clinical observations on man were correct. Without the help of Mrs. H. Blackman ("Mrs. Bee") of the same Department, this chance would have been lost irretrievably. Mr. Donald Nisbet, my wartime comrade-in-arms, was at all times most helpful in checking the manuscripts of my work, and Dr. Royal Lee, Head of the Lee Foundation for Nutritional Research, made it possible for me to have "The Drama of Fluorine" published. To all of them I extend my sincere thanks.

Leo Spira, M.D., Ph.D. (Med.)

344 West 72nd Street
New York 23, New York
December 1953

Table of Contents

[Editor's Note Regarding Modern Usage:

fluorine: [fluo·rine, | flʊərin] (noun) **fluoride**

Fluorine as used by the author is completely synonymous and interchangeable with our daily use of the word fluoride, as in fluoride toothpaste. It is also the additive used in the controversial practice of municipal water fluoridation.

The terms fluorine and fluoride, in nearly all medical and news articles, are interchangeable. In the field of chemistry there is a clear distinction, but it does not apply to normal usage.

Other term definitions are found in the Glossary at the end of this book.]

Chapter 1: What Is The Matter With These People

When in 1922 I went to live and practise in London, England, I found that many of my patients, whatever the original complaint for which they came to consult me, upon inquiry also complained of certain troubles which, taken together, seemed to constitute a uniform pattern of an unfamiliar disease. That the general occurrence of these symptoms was not wholly fortuitous did not occur to me until after a year of close study.

Amongst these symptoms an outstanding feature was obstinate constipation lasting variable periods of time, between two or three days in milder cases and up to as many as seven days at a stretch in more pronounced ones. Surprisingly enough, people appeared to take constipation as a matter of course, as something that did not count as an abnormality, especially when it was handed down from generation to generation. (If they had ever mentioned constipation to their medical adviser, not as a serious trouble, but as a minor ailment, he had brushed it aside as something quite irrelevant and unimportant, since, in his experience, it was so widespread and common amongst the population at large that it had to be considered as normal rather than exceptional in the life of mankind.) To bolster up this explanation, which even in his own mind was anything but convincing, the medical adviser would assure his patient that in no medical textbook had he ever come across a statement to the effect that man's bowels should move every day. Against such an argument, one supported by the authority of medical textbooks, there was obviously no appeal whatsoever. The judgment was final: Habitual constipation was something from which you did not die; you had it just as most other people had, and you must put up with it. The condition was not harmful, but should it ever trouble you or offend your fussy belief that your inside must be kept in a clean condition, well, what was wrong with any of the numerous kinds of pills, tablets, oils, and what not, on the market? A packet of good old Epsom — or Glauber — salts would only cost you sixpence, so take them every day, or as often as you felt you needed them.

Since many people, probably the great majority of the population, do feel that their insides should be kept as clean as their outsides, whatever the opinion of their medical adviser, and since they are often troubled by the discomfort of constipation lasting several days at a time, a good number did acquire the habit of taking aperients and laxatives of one kind or another. For them, helping the bowels became part of their daily routine. Many of them denied that they were constipated; they would, they said, not allow themselves to be constipated, so they took Epsom — or Glauber — salts every morning. Thus, there came into being a nation with the unenviable reputation of a constipated nation, on which there flourished a tremendous industry engaged in the manufacture of "opening medicines". There was no longer any need to consult the doctor for mere constipation, and the numerous chemist's shops, drug stores, etc., springing up at the corner of every block, were there to remind the public that these pills, or those tablets, medicines, salts, oils, etc., would do them, the general public, a lot of good, and to assure them that, just to help suffering humanity, these remedies, worth double the amount, would be charged at only half the price.

Constipation was not an isolated symptom. It soon became obvious that it was accompanied by severe flatulence, an excessive gas formation sometimes so pronounced that the victims — man, woman or child — looked as if they were in an advanced stage of pregnancy. There was a young girl, not sophisticated either bodily or mentally, who, whilst serving in the army during the last World War, was accused by the other girls in the camp of being pregnant. When by the order of her commanding officer she came to be examined, she immediately said, "I know, sir, the reason why I have to be examined, but I am not pregnant. It is my stomach, which goes up and down, up and down, several times a day." The girl was not pregnant; she was suffering from excessive gas formation in her bowels.

Gas formation has to be relieved somehow or other. Belching and retching is one method of relief; another is "passing wind" down the bowel with results sometimes distressing alike to the sufferer and to those around him, especially when the gas has to find an outlet at a social gathering. The victim of this complaint is naturally given a wide berth on account of his "bad manners".

If not relieved, the bowel distension and the constipation would sometimes cause attacks of colicky pain of such severity that the family doctor would be called in, and occasionally the acute pain and the accompanying rigidity of the abdominal wall led him to the perfectly justifiable conclusion that the case might be one of an abdominal emergency — of acute appendicitis requiring immediate operation, of an attack of gall-stones or of a stone in the kidney, to be relieved only by an injection of morphia, or of ptomaine poisoning. It has, however, often enough been reported that when in such circumstances an operation had been performed, no pathology could be detected. Subsequently, in spite of the operation, the attacks of pain recurred.

Changes in the mouth were frequently found. Small blisters formed on the mucous membrane, which broke down to turn into ulcers and cracks, and caused great pain on eating and talking. Gingivitis was a regular feature, the gums appearing red, inflamed, swollen and bleeding. Sometimes a condition developed which was identical with pyorrhoea and. caused the teeth to become loose so that they had to be extracted and be replaced by artificial dentures. I have seen children in their teens wearing complete sets of upper and lower dentures.

Changes in the hair and nails were also observed. The finger nails were so brittle that even a slight accidental knock on a hard object, for example the edge of a table, caused them to break across. Sometimes they were described as being so soft as to be easily torn at their free edges. Often transverse thickened elevations of varied width alternated with shallow depressions across the upper surface of the finger and toe nails, and gave them a furrowed appearance. When allowed to grow beyond the tips of the fingers and toes, the nails tended to curl round them in a claw-like or beak-like fashion. In a few cases there was a loosening of a toe nail without the slightest warning, even to the extent of its being lifted out of its bed and falling off. The commonest feature, however, was the occurrence of raised longitudinal ridges on the surface of the finger and toe nails. They could easily be seen as well as felt on a cut portion of such a nail. In one case, these longitudinal ridges were so pronounced that their owner boasted that he was able to strike a match on them. In addition, dull, opaque, chalky-white specks, patches or transverse bands, such as are familiar to everybody, appeared frequently on several nails. Toe nails, especially those on the big toes, often showed a permanent discoloration, the colour being a dull mixture in which dark grey and brown of variable intensity preponderated.

There was a frequent complaint that the hair was falling out prematurely with the result that some men, not yet 20 years old, could easily be taken to be past middle age. Such changes in the nails and hair, unless rapidly progressing to a state seriously affecting the personal appearance, only rarely led the victim to seek medical advice. The medical man, finding no visible cause for the pronounced loss of hair, would, more likely than not, refer him to the probability of identical ancestral trouble and remark unconcernedly that there was nothing that could be done about it. In despair the victim would often turn to quack remedies offered him by the barber — whose own skilfully made wig could not hide the fact that he himself belonged to the category of bald men.

Things took a much more serious turn if, in due course, one of these patients developed a skin disease. What a skin disease implies is known only to one who has been afflicted himself. In most cases, it is perhaps not so much the physical as the mental suffering of the patient that makes his life well-nigh unbearable. A disease of widespread occurrence is "athlete's foot", which is characterized by the development of blisters between and underneath the toes, causing intense itching and burning. It is generally attributed to a fungus infection, because in some cases a fungus has been detected under the microscope, although in many other cases none can ever be found. The application of an ointment would be prescribed, which would destroy the epidermis and any fungus with it. To prevent re-infection of the skin through the wearing apparel, believed to be likewise infected, shoes, socks, and everything that might have come in contact with the affected foot would be ordered to be burned or disinfected. If, when the effect of the ointment has worn off, the regenerated epidermis showed signs of recurrence, the blame would be put on the inefficient disinfection of the wearing apparel. With each recurrence the procedure would be repeated, until the patient, now thoroughly wearied, would try to make the best of it and bear patiently with his foot trouble for the rest of his life.

Some people would complain of itching in different parts of the body without any underlying cause being visible. At social parties, ladies in beautiful evening dresses exposing their back down the spine were occasionally seen to be scratching with the aid of an antique long-handled

3

"back scratcher" in the form of a carved ivory hand with fingers half-bent, employed in earlier times to obtain relief from intense irritation of the skin; or a friendly neighbour at the dining table would be asked to lend a hand to scratch the not easily accessible part of the back.

In other cases, recurrent attacks of boils or weals would cause invalidism for a variable length of time. Worse still, eczema with all its grievous consequences, sometimes developed anywhere on the body. If resistent to treatment carried out at home, hospital treatment would sometimes be necessitated, especially when the eczema had affected a large part of the body. A painter's brush would be dipped into the pot containing the ointment or lotion believed to be capable of curing the skin disease, and liberally applied. The application sometimes proved too strong, as evidenced by the development of an additional inflammatory dermatitis, and then another and yet another ointment or lotion would be tried out, occasionally with soothing effect.

Many of these patients would complain of neuralgiae in the arms and legs, or of cramps in the calves occurring mainly at night during sleep and causing them much alarm. The affected calf feels stone-hard during the cramp, which lasts for a minute or two and then gradually eases leaving a dull pain behind. Attacks of pain in various joints, especially in the wrist and fingers and in the ankle and instep were frequently complained of and hiccup, vehement sneezing, "running nose", lachrymation, salivation and frequent attacks of "common cold" were also encountered. The patient often said that he suffered from "pins and needles" in the hands and fingers, and to a lesser extent in his feet and toes, and from a sensation of deadness and numbness, which, he had been informed, was due to poor blood circulation. As a rule his blood pressure was low.

Generally, such patients appeared to lead a wretched existence. They felt apprehensive and irritable and were subject to frequent attacks of depression and even melancholia with loss of energy and general lassitude. Their outlook on life was gloomy, and without good reason, they expected a disaster of one kind or another to occur at any moment. There were periods when they felt well, but the persistence of certain disabilities would remind them that, as on previous occasions, their symptoms would probably recur.

It must, of course, not be assumed that all the symptoms were in each case developed to the marked degree which has been described, or that they ran concurrently in every patient. In some patients a few of, or even all, the symptoms might be observed at the same time. In others, certain symptoms predominated, the digestive trouble, or the skin disease or the mental disturbances prevailing over the others.

As time went on, the idea began to crystallize in my mind that the disease might be due to some kind of chronic poisoning, and since a disturbance of the digestive canal always formed part of the picture to a greater or lesser extent, it was suspected that some kind of food might be at the root of the trouble. The food would obviously have to be such as was most indispensable in everyday life, for those suffering from the symptom-complex belonged to different spheres of society. Bread and its ingredients,

4

meat, milk, butter, vegetables, fruit, tea and coffee, sugar, salt and drinking water had to be considered.

In an endeavour to find out which of these articles might be the offending factor in the cases of various patients, one article of food after another was struck off the list of diet, and it was recommended that water should be taken only after being boiled. The results, however, were in each case negative, and it was concluded that experiments in this direction were fruitless.

Chapter 2: I Turn Into A Research Worker

My endeavour to find a common factor responsible for this symptom-complex affecting large sections of the population thus seemed in danger of failure. Fate now came to my assistance at an opportune moment. Paradoxically, it was my good fortune that I myself, hitherto enjoying perfect health, became a victim to the disease. This gave me a welcome opportunity to study the problem with precision. Self-observation, as objective and reliable as I could make it, helped me to eliminate such symptoms described by patients as appeared to be inaccurate or misleading. To obtain a clear picture of their several complaints, it was necessary to separate the wheat from the chaff.

Since the disease took a chronic course from the start, it was impossible to determine its insidious onset with any degree of accuracy. It seems certain, however, that the first symptoms to appear are digestive disturbances, but they are usually overlooked or attributed to some transitory attack of indigestion. It soon becomes obvious that they are steadily progressing towards a chronic condition, even if care is exercised in the diet. The first visible manifestation of something being radically amiss is in some cases the appearance of cutaneous changes between and underneath the toes. Intense burning and itching follows, and this indicates that the condition known as "athlete's foot" is developed fully; this condition is not likely ever to disappear altogether without treatment aimed at the elimination of the hypothetical poison.

In some cases, without any previous warning, an eczema makes its appearance on and between the fingers, spreading gradually towards the wrists. It is said to be an extension of the fungous infection from the "athlete's foot", but in most cases no fungus can be detected microscopically in that locality either. The skin over the fingers burns and itches as much as the skin between the toes, and, since the victim does not yet realize what is in store for him, he hopefully applies the various ointments or lotions to the skin, which he covers by bandages as prescribed by his dermatologist. He does not worry very much at first, believing that the applications will soon cure the disease. As time goes on, however, his hopes are replaced by despondency. The treatment having failed to improve the trouble, X-rays and radium are applied to destroy the non-existent fungus. Months pass by, and the patient is by now in a state of despair, his hands still having to be covered by bandages. If the patient is a medical man his lot is all the heavier, for he is confronted

7

with the prospect of having to give up his profession altogether. In the meantime, a year, a long-drawn out year, has gone, but there is not the slightest sign of improvement.

It was at this juncture that for some reason or other I entered what in England is considered to be a sanctuary reserved for the cook. As spotlessly clean as her kitchen, the cook was just at work preparing dinner. On the kitchen table pots and pans were spread out, the very aluminium cooking utensils which I had bought some short time previously on account of their attractive appearance. The shop assistant was so pleasantly insistent that they were the best that money could buy, and, in particular, were very economical in fuel because of their light weight, that I could not resist purchasing them, although I personally had never seen aluminium utensils in use before.

When I saw on the table my once so bright and shiny aluminium cooking utensils, half-filled with water to which some article of food or other was to be added, I had the horrid suspicion that cook was perhaps not the model of cleanliness I had always believed her to be. Horrified, I asked her why she allowed the pots to become as unsightly looking as they did, but she calmly explained that aluminium cooking utensils always changed colour, turning pink, red, mauve, blue and black, assuming on other occasions a bright silvery appearance. It all depended, she said, on what kind of food was cooked in them at the time. Apple sauce and rhubarb turn dark green, if left standing in an aluminium dish. Cranberries turn from bright red to black, and potatoes have dark streaks in them when boiled in an aluminium pot. When tap water is boiled in an aluminium kettle, the inside turns grey to black. Tomatoes boiled in an aluminium pan make it look clean and bright, in the same way as soda or soap does.

The cook's explanation sounded so honest that I was disarmed and my confidence fully restored, but suddenly it occurred to me: "Good Heavens! Can it be that this is the cause of the eczema on my hands and fingers, and of my athlete's foot? Is it possible that food prepared in aluminium cooking utensils is the culprit for which I was so eagerly looking, a cause of the disease that affects large sections of the population?"

A lengthy conference with cook followed, from which it transpired that to keep aluminium cooking utensils clean, soda, or a material containing soda, such as soap, special cleaning powders, etc., are used. Treated in this way, they assume a bright and shiny appearance. It is obvious that this process is the result of corrosion, the superficial layer of the metal being removed by the cleaning material each time it is employed. Since aluminium is readily soluble

8

in both acid and alkaline media, such as are present in food which is being cooked, it does not call for an undue stretch of the imagination to conclude that, by the corroding effect of the ingredients, the metal must be dissolved and contaminate the food.

It is a strange sensation for any medical man to treat a disease of his own. It is never practised when a more than transitory indisposition is concerned. In my case, however, there was no alternative: I had either to help myself or to give up my profession. To be perfectly frank, by this time I was deeply concerned about my future and my medical career. Something would have to be done for my fingers and hands, which still had to be constantly covered with bandages. The procedure I intended to adopt was in the first instance to experiment on my own body. I was going to turn myself into a combined research worker and a guinea pig. In my research I would have perfect freedom of action, unencumbered by any preconceived theories concerning the fungous origin of a number of skin diseases, including my own.

The proposed work seemed quite simple. The question was: Had or had not food prepared in aluminium cooking utensils anything to do with my skin trouble? For the sake of experiment, the aluminium kitchen utensils were not removed altogether from the household, but the order was given that instead of their being cleaned with soda only water and brush were to be employed. To absorb and to eliminate the poison accumulated in the body, large doses of charcoal and an aperient were taken. Every kind of local treatment was discontinued. This resulted, within a few days, in bringing the hitherto rebellious skin affection on the hand and fingers, as well as on the toes, to a standstill. The angry-looking, inflamed and sore skin quietened down, and the steadily progressing deterioration of the condition was halted. The burning and itching on the hands and feet were at the same time considerably relieved.

This was indeed a promising start and my despondency vanished. The aluminium utensils were now removed altogether, and this resulted in a further improvement of the condition. There could now be no doubt that all the symptoms were due to a poison contained in the cooking utensils.

For sake of accuracy it must be here stated that, although the cutaneous manifestations had finally disappeared altogether, the gastro-intestinal symptoms, albeit considerably alleviated, persisted in appearing shortly after meals. The possibility of the presence of an irritant in other sources had therefore to be pursued, possible sources being drinking water and canned foods.

I have already remarked that drinking water had been under suspicion for some time, and that I had recommended that it should be ingested only after being boiled. This procedure, however, had no effect at all on the course of the disease. A more energetic measure was therefore decided upon. Ingestion of tap water was now stopped altogether, and it was replaced by a pure and wholesome natural mineral water, which was also used for boiling food wherever possible. A diet was chosen which excluded everything prepared in tap water. Only fresh fruit, or fruit and potatoes baked in their jackets, soft-boiled eggs, etc., were to be taken.

This regime was applied with the strictest perseverance in all the cases suspected as being due to a poison derived from the sources mentioned. A complete cure, not obtainable by any of the many methods of treatment hitherto applied, was maintained as long as the patients persevered with the regime prescribed. They were gradually put on an ordinary diet, but were not allowed to use aluminium cooking utensils, tap water or any other likely sources of contamination, and they remained perfectly well as long as they took small doses of charcoal and an aperient. In cases in which for some reason they omitted these precautions, however, the symptoms again made their appearance, only to disappear as rapidly as before when the regime was again strictly followed.

It is not proposed to illustrate any individual cases which suffered from chronic poisoning, without involvement of the skin, by the irritant contained in aluminium cooking utensils, in tap water, in canned food, etc. Their number was very large and, while in general conforming to the above description, they presented a varying degree of sensitiveness to the irritant. Illustration of these cases is omitted since it might be suggested by sceptical critics that the cure claimed in such cases of longstanding gastro-intestinal trouble was due to psychological effects. It may, however, be accepted as a fact that all these cases improved within a very short time, often not exceeding a few weeks after the commencement of the treatment.

The absolute correctness of the conclusions arrived at cannot be demonstrated more clearly than by citing one or two cases of patients who exhibited predominantly cutaneous manifestations of a systemic disease, in addition to the other signs of the symptom-complex. As a matter of fact, the digestive trouble in some of these cases was relatively slight and was often overlooked by the patients, owing to their preoccupation with the condition of the skin.

I was urged to treat a child who had infantile eczema on the face and all over the body, for which every conceivable remedy had been tried in vain. It was useless for me to protest that I am not a dermatologist. The distressed mother stated that little Alan, aged 5, had had the skin trouble for 4½ years and always had to be kept covered with bandages. On account of the rash the child could never be shown even to relatives or close friends. He used to fall asleep from sheer exhaustion, but would wake up again at frequent intervals.

It was all very well for me to say that I was not a dermatologist, and that I had never, even in my hospital days, seen a skin disease as bad as this one, and that consequently I was not justified in even attempting treatment where all skin specialists have failed. The condition of the child was so pitiable that I decided something had to be done.

I began by explaining to the disconsolate mother that, although I had got rid of my own skin trouble, I had no means of judging whether by an identical method of treatment I could do the poor child any good. I was willing to try, however, for even if I failed, I would not be the first to fail and no harm would be done by the attempt. This time there was no experimenting. Orders were given how to proceed, and it was impressed upon the mother and nurse that my instructions were to be followed meticulously. No insistence on this point was necessary, however, for where a sufferer from a protracted skin trouble is concerned any directions which might contribute towards the alleviation of the suffering will be followed implicitly.

After 10 weeks' systemic treatment, without any local applications whatsoever, the child was completely cured. He remained entirely free from the eczema for 2½ years, when the mother, believing the child now out of danger of susceptibility, gave him food not subjected to the various restrictions, and the condition recurred. On resumption of the treatment the skin healed again.

Very soon another mother was asking for help. Her child, June, aged 11, had been suffering from infantile eczema, diagnosed as of allergic nature, practically since birth. The skin was even then unusually dry, and the medical man in attendance thought the child would probably never have a normal skin. The actual eczema made its appearance at the age of one month. Continuous local treatment suggested by different dermatologists proved ineffective and the child had to be kept permanently in bandages. In fact, for some years splints had to be used, on medical orders, to prevent her from scratching. The local applications succeeded in alleviating the intense irritation only for a short time. Apart from such short intervals, the misery of the child's life, and that of the family, was said to be beyond description.

Identical treatment was begun and every kind of local application discarded. In 5 weeks the child was practically cured.

11

Chapter 3: The Culprit Is Cornered

In accordance with medical tradition, the medical man is in the first instance required to alleviate or, if possible, to cure the condition troubling his patient. He is guided by the knowledge acquired in the course of his training, at lectures and demonstrations, as well as from medical textbooks. As time progresses, he enlarges his knowledge by experience gained first in the hospital ward and later in his own independent work. In medicine, just as in every other field of human activity, the more experience he has acquired the better will be his clinical judgment. It is not for him, however, to deviate from what has been laid down in current medical textbooks, even though he knows that only rarely do they contain anything startlingly novel, since in the great majority of cases they originated not at the bedside in the hospital ward but in the medical library, where a number of older textbooks are at hand to serve as a basis for writing new ones.

Nor is the medical man in a position to do anything but pursue in his daily work the beaten track generally accepted by his contemporaries. If he has an independent mind and tries to put his own ideas into practise he will soon be branded as a crank by his less progressive professional brethren, as well as by the public. In addition, neither the average medical man nor the average patient can often afford the time and money required to go deeper into the cause of a complicated illness. It is so much simpler to make use of one of the innumerable remedies supplied by the chemical industry. It cannot, of course, be denied that by this, mainly empirical, approach to medical problems in recent years a certain amount of progress has been achieved. Nor will it be denied that important discoveries have been made, particularly in the field of physiology, thus laying the foundation for further advance in medical knowledge. On the other hand, it must be affirmed that on the whole Medicine, as at present practised in everyday life, has made only limited headway.

Conditions are even less favourable where Preventive Medicine is concerned. In the course of his studies the young student had only very limited opportunity to concentrate on studying how to prevent disease. If he wished to devote his full time to this subject, the graduate would embark on a new course of study in the field of Hygiene and Preventive Medicine. After completion of the course his work would confine him to a governmental office where, as a competent civil servant, he would deal mainly with statistics concerning the incidence and prevention of infectious diseases.

Generally speaking, relatively few in the profession, namely, those who are in the privileged position of being financially independent, can aspire to set out on an organized search for the causation of disease as it occurs in everyday life. There are some, however, who in spite of all difficulties find themselves impelled to persevere in the pursuit of truth.

Having arrived at the conclusion that the favourable outcome of the treatment of my own eczema and of the eczema of the two children, as well as of several other cases of severe skin disease that followed, was indeed due not to psychological effects but to the removal of the still unidentified irritant ingested daily with food and drink, I considered it my duty, in accordance with the idealistic teachings inculcated in us by our elders in the course of our medical training, to write out a report on my observations for submission to the medical profession. This, we used to be told, was the procedure to be adopted in cases which we thought of sufficient interest to be worth communicating. The paper submitted was entitled: "Some skin manifestations and their relation to the disturbance of the gastro-intestinal tract" and, it was soon followed by another one reporting; on "Chronic poisoning by an irritant contained in aluminium cooking utensils and tap water". Both were dated 1926. Having as yet had no experience of the way in which certain medical journals dealt with contributions to medical knowledge, I had no doubt that my papers would be regarded as of great importance and accepted for publication. Surely, I could not be the only medical man who was daily confronted with signs and symptoms of this unnamed disease picture prevalent amongst the population at large. Many others amongst my professional brethren must have often enough been puzzled by the simultaneous occurrence of apparently incongruous features of a morbid condition, for which no explanation could be found in any of the medical textbooks. To my simple mind, it seemed the duty of the journal, rather than its favour bestowed on me, to accept and to publish without delay what I was reporting. Instead, after several months passed, I learnt that my work was rejected. I could not understand it at all. Was there anything radically wrong with the style of my writing? I did not think so. Or was I, at the age of 40, too young to point out to my profession that there was something radically wrong somewhere, when patients, who have long been sufferers from certain skin diseases, could obtain no relief from their suffering by the older methods of treatment, but were in a relatively short time cured by methods attacking the trouble from the inside of the body? Possibly! Or, in addition to this was it perhaps heresy, incriminating aluminium cooking utensils, which kept so beautifully shiny so long as they were cleaned with soda, or with materials containing soda, or to suggest that there might be something wrong with our tap water, the best drinking water in the world? I wondered. It seemed as if sufferers were condemned to keep their skin diseases and certain other diseases for a long time, perhaps even for the rest of their lives. So no medical man was even to try to lighten medical darkness: "What was good enough for our grandfathers is good enough for us."

It was, however, not good enough for me. I knocked at the doors of other medical journals, but the result was always the same. It occurred to me that I might be luckier if instead of proceeding the direct way I invited the help of an influential member of my profession. I soon gave up this idea, however, for my pride kept me from using oblique methods of approach. My ambition was by now in danger of being replaced by bewilderment, hopelessness, despondency and disgust.

There lived at that time a celebrated surgeon, whose name was on the lips of everybody in the profession. In his younger days he certainly made some very valuable contributions towards improved technique in surgery. At a later stage of his career, however, he formed the unfortunate opinion that cancer, which frequently affects an infected large intestine, could be prevented by removing the large intestine altogether. The results of the operation, which he performed for a number of years, proved deplorable, and he discarded the idea. The hitherto radically-minded surgeon developed into an ardent advocate of more conservative surgery. After being exposed to ridicule, he now became a target for the contempt of his professional brethren. Having admitted his past errors of surgical judgment, he was now ostracized because of his more conservative outlook on life. His attempts to justify himself were refused publication, and, understandably enough, he became embittered and cynical, feeding his grudge against the medical powers that be.

Someone suggested I should go and see him, and ask for his advice, for to some extent we were both in the same boat, although his position, both socially and professionally, was immeasurably higher than I could ever expect mine to be. When I was admitted into the great man's presence, I was greeted by a few kind words of consolation. He seemed to understand my predicament completely and he sent me to the editor of a little monthly journal who, he said, would publish what I so ardently wished the profession to know. When I left a few minutes later I was a much happier man, now that I was assured that my two papers would appear in print. True, the monthly was as obscure as I was, but I felt that the ice was broken. It later occurred to me that perhaps my sponsor himself had founded the little journal, so as to have a platform from which he could ventilate his own grievances. Be that as it might, I was pleased to feel that the fact that my two articles were being published might one day help to facilitate the publication of further articles based on my observations.

I spoke to anybody who was prepared to listen to my story. Only a few were interested. Amongst them was a dentist, who informed me that one of his medical friends would like to read the manuscripts of my two papers, although they had not yet appeared in print. I regained my courage and determination. Here at last was one medical man who was interested in my work on the deleterious effect of ingestion of food prepared in aluminium cooking utensils and of tap water! My manuscripts were returned in due course with a few words of appreciation. With the subsequent appearance of my papers in print in 1928, my battle seemed to have been won at long last, at least for the time being. What was printed under my name nobody could ever take away from me. I realized soon enough, however, that my publications would not make the slightest impression anywhere outside the little monthly journal.

The dentist's medical friend turned out to be quite a shrewd fellow. My manuscripts seem to have impressed him as being interesting, at any rate as far as food prepared in aluminium cooking utensils was concerned. He thereupon wrote a paper of his own, based on mine, and submitted it for publication first to one medical journal, then to another. When it met with the same fate as my papers, he had it published independently in the form of a monograph describing the danger of food contaminated by aluminium. I learned later that as many copies of the monograph were printed as there were medical men in the country, each of whom received a copy with the compliments of the author. I myself obtained one in a roundabout way.

It will be seen that I was learning quite a lot about medical journalism. This was how medical research was being carried out and its results brought to the notice of the medical profession!

A few years passed after the publication of my two papers, and they did not seem to have made any difference to the world and everything continued just as before. My study of the problem of chronic poisoning by an irritant contaminating everyday articles of food and drink also continued, however. The next thing to be determined was the identity of the poison.

Amongst the various signs and symptoms of the poisoning, the sensation of "pins and needles" and of numbness in fingers and hands was frequently complained of. I was told that this sensation was attributed to anaemia and to deficient blood circulation. At this juncture fate once more came to my assistance for I myself now experienced this complaint on frequent occasions.

I observed that the fingers mainly affected were the little finger and the adjacent surface of the ring finger. As a medical man I knew that this area is supplied by fibres of a certain nerve, called the ulnar nerve, which comes down the arm and forearm and terminates in the 1½ fingers here mentioned, just as the remaining 3½ digits of the hand are supplied by another nerve, called the radial nerve, which comes down on the other side of the arm and forearm. I also happened to remember that there is only one poison which attacks the ulnar nerve, namely, fluorine, just as lead attacks the radial nerve. I thus realized that it might be fluorine, and the defective blood circulation, which was responsible for the sensation of numbness in the fingers. It looked as if I had arrived at the threshold of an important discovery.

Should my supposition prove to be correct, the all-important question would be: How did fluorine find its way into the body? A reply to this question would be all the more difficult to give since fluorine (unlike chlorine, iodine and bromine, to which it is chemically closely related) has had little attention paid to it, apart from cursory mention in textbooks used by students of Medicine and Chemistry. If the results of my search for the cause of that hitherto obscure illness (which 1 had traced back to food prepared in aluminium cooking utensils and to drinking water) were substantiated, then obviously it would have to be assumed that the fluorine was derived from these two sources. I, therefore, now concentrated all my attention on this chemical substance.

As time progressed, I felt more and more uneasy about the procedure by which the contents of my two papers had been adopted as the basis for a monograph that purported to be original work. Owing to its circulation amongst the medical profession, the monograph was likely to be widely accepted as the fruit of original research. If left unchallenged, it would acquire undeserved priority, a possibility that I could not tolerate. More important still, however, my belief that fluorine might play an essential part in further research demanded immediate action.

I therefore applied to the Hampstead Branch of the British Medical Association for a meeting to be arranged, at which I proposed to read a paper on "Chronic poisoning by an irritant contained in tap water and cooking utensils, producing skin manifestations and gastro-intestinal disturbances". As meetings at which medical subjects were discussed were rare events at that Branch, there was no difficulty in having my application approved. I did not really anticipate a large attendance, but the number of medical men who did come to listen to what I had to say was far beyond my expectations. Amongst the audience was my dentist friend and his medical friend with his numerous followers.

I spoke at some length and laid special emphasis on the possibility that fluorine might be an important clue in the search for the cause of the obscure disease. At the end of my address, of course, I did not fail to acknowledge the help given by my colleague in publishing the results of my work.

The chairman's frequent glances at his watch during the course of my address did not deter me in the slightest. I was gratified with the long discussion that followed and with the suggestion made by one of those present that, in view of the number who desired to participate in the discussion during the short time available, a second meeting should be arranged. The second meeting never materialized. Nor would the chairman comply with my request that, in accordance with custom, he should send a report on the meeting to the British Medical Journal, the official weekly organ of the British Medical Association. The report, he said, would have to come from me. In view of my past experience I did not bother. For the time being I was quite satisfied that through the meeting I had achieved what my two papers published in the little medical monthly could never have achieved, namely, that the subject of my work had come to the notice of a medical public, however limited in numbers.

A further development followed the week after the meeting, when a short letter to the editor appeared in the widely read British Medical Journal, drawing attention to what I had said at the meeting concerning the toxic action of fluorine on man. In response I wrote a letter in which I further emphasized the deleterious effect of this potent poison.

Everything seemed to be developing favourably. Truth could not be suppressed for long, in spite of vested interests. I felt that, whilst the time was not yet ripe for any suggestion that the quality of what was still generally believed to be the best drinking water in the world was not all that it ought to be, my warning against the use of aluminium cooking utensils was gradually being heeded by the housewife, who was now becoming conscious of the way in which the appearance of the metal changed during the process of preparing food. The average medical man, however, would more often than not refuse to budge an inch from his narrow path of prescribing a medicine for the leading symptom complained of by his patient; an attempt to prevent the development of that symptom was not yet part of his medical philosophy. It became obvious that his attention had to be drawn to the existence of an evil in a more direct way, by means of a frontal attack. The result of any discussion within a few isolated

18

medical circles, concerning the deleterious effect of food prepared in aluminium kitchen utensils, which might result from one meeting, however successful, and from one or two short letters to the editor of a medical journal was, in the absence of more serious attention on the part of the medical profession, bound soon to die a natural death. It was necessary to awaken the interest of the whole medical profession in the harmful effect of fluorine, if further evidence of the presence of this element in aluminium cooking utensils, so far assumed on the basis of clinical observation, was to be obtained.

A study of the manufacture of aluminium kitchen utensils followed. It was carried out in technical libraries in an atmosphere utterly different from that encountered in purely medical research. Temporarily transformed into a student of metallurgy, I acquired a better insight into the mechanism of my objective. In the manufacture of the aluminium metal two indispensable raw materials are employed, namely, bauxite, which is an aluminium mineral, and cryolite, a fluorine mineral. Even after purification, both of them contain various impurities. Alumina, which chemically is an aluminium oxide derived from the bauxite, is placed in the furnace, where it is dissolved in the liquid bath of cryolite. A strong electric current is passed through the bath and the dissociation of alumina into aluminium and oxygen is effected.

The product so obtained appears on the market as "primary" aluminium, and this is graded according to the amount of impurities present. Amongst the chief impurities are iron, copper, silicon, lead and tin. The "primary" metal is made into aluminium sheets, and used for the manufacture of kitchen utensils.

Scraps of the metal recovered in the course of the manufacture are again remelted, but no further refining is practicable. Consequently, this "secondary" metal contains more impurities than does the "primary" product, chief among them being, in addition to those present in the "primary" product, manganese, zinc, arsenic and antimony. This "secondary" aluminium is likewise used in the production of kitchen utensils.

Moreover, for the manufacture of cooking utensils, alloys of either the "primary" or the "secondary" aluminium are produced. The possible number of aluminium alloys is almost limitless, and includes those with silicon, copper, iron, magnesium, nickel, tin, zinc, or combinations of these metals.

When considering the deleterious effects of food prepared in aluminium cooking utensils, we are thus confronted not with one but with several poisons. That the metal gradually corrodes every housewife knows, as has already been pointed out. As a result of this corrosion, both the components of the metal and their inevitable impurities are set free, so as to contaminate the food. Contrary to irresponsible statements made in certain quarters, the element aluminium itself is a potent poison. It has been classed in one group together with copper, arsenic and lead by several outstanding investigators in this country as well as on the Continent of Europe. The high toxicity of the other components of the aluminium alloys and of their several impurities is too well known to require further elaboration. The role played by cryolite as a source of contamination by fluorine has, however, not been fully appreciated.

Chapter 4: The Aluminium Industry Turns Vindictive

Co-ordinating the knowledge gathered from the medical investigation on the one hand and from the metallurgical study of the manufacture of aluminium on the other, thus promised to be fruitful. The as yet unsubstantiated clinical incrimination of fluorine as a probable contaminant of food prepared in aluminium kitchen utensils was now materially strengthened by the fact that this poison was contained in cryolite, which plays a prominent part in the process of their manufacture, as well as by the physical characteristics of the metal. The belief that the use of aluminium cooking utensils was detrimental to health ceased to be a myth, an illusory outgrowth of imagination. Instead, it became a working hypothesis, henceforth to be relentlessly pursued. It was enthusiastically accepted by all those who had long suffered, or whose children and friends had suffered, from intractable skin diseases that would not respond to any of the numerous recognized methods of local treatment, and who now benefitted by the new conception of the cause of their trouble. They were soon joined by others, who became converts to the idea of treating the cause of their digestive disorders by giving up their aluminium pots and pans rather than by regularly taking their "opening medicines" and pills and tablets of various kinds, which they had carried with them for use in the course of the day whilst away from home. It was no longer necessary for them to lead the life of invalids.

Nevertheless, the hope that the study of the problem would ever be taken up by those competent to investigate remained as remote as ever. It was not to be expected that the vast majority of medical men would change their preconceived ideas, for the simple reason that they had their hands full of work the whole time, pursuing the daily routine of everyday Medicine. In addition, it had to be conceded that the relatively few in the medical profession who were carrying out research work along their chosen path of interest could not be expected to deviate from their particular object of study, on which they might have been working for many years and which would most likely occupy their full time and energy for the rest of their lives, in the hope that the result of their work would in due course contribute towards improved health.

The medical man who happens to hit upon an original and hitherto entirely unknown subject, however important that subject may turn out to be, has to rely upon his own wits. His is the difficult task of the pioneer, without whose enthusiasm, perseverance and hard work no progress will ever be made. Having laid the foundation for further work, he now concentrates on trying to increase the number of those who might one day become associated with it, by adding brick upon brick for building up the edifice. There was, so far, not the slightest indication that the medical press, to whose sphere of activities the matter primarily belonged, would recommend further investigation. It therefore became necessary somehow or other to circumvent the apathy of those who aspired to be looked upon as the custodians of medical knowledge and progress, and to act independently. There seemed to be no alternative to adopting the method applied by my medical friend, who had tried to interest the profession in the deleterious effect of food prepared in aluminium cooking utensils. A monograph incorporating the contents of my two papers, to which my recent findings concerning the role played by fluorine were added, was compiled under the title: "The Clinical Aspect of Chronic Poisoning by Aluminium and Its Alloys". A foreword by my great teacher the pharmacologist Hans Horst Meyer of Vienna University, added considerable weight to the importance of the work. Many years previously another of his pupils had written an important thesis on the toxicity of the element long before aluminium was used for culinary purposes.

Sixty thousand copies of the monograph were printed and a copy sent to each medical man in the country with the author's compliments. Although I personally delivered them at one of the central post offices in bundles of several hundreds at a time, many copies mysteriously disappeared and never arrived at their destination. Numerous letters appreciating the importance of the work poured in from the recipients, but not a single notice appeared in the columns of any of the various British medical journals, although they, too, were supplied with a copy each. For reasons best known to themselves, the monograph had to be ignored and open discussion of it discouraged. By contrast, a large number of leading medical journals on the Continent of Europe published extensive reviews, urging the necessity for further investigation. On one occasion a man, introducing himself as a journalist strongly opposed to the use of aluminium in the kitchen, came to see me in connection with my work. He asked me for further details of my investigation. I showed him all my laboratory reports on numerous patients who were suffering from the effects of food prepared in aluminium pots and pans. At the conclusion of our discussion, he asked me to lend him all these reports which he would, he said, utilize in his forthcoming publication and return to me in the course of the next few days. When they were not returned, I wrote him a letter to his stated address, but the letter came back with the remark of the post office that no such man was living there.

Whilst the medical press was thus still standing aloof letting things take their course, the public, realizing that it was their battle which was being fought for them, sent in letters to the editor of the national paper, "The Times", requesting that the matter should be brought to the attention of responsible quarters. In due course, an editorial appeared in that influential daily suggesting that, in view of the misgivings of the average British housewife, an inter-governmental committee should be set up to determine whether aluminium cooking utensils were or were not harmful for the use in the kitchen. Just as in the past, however, when those opposed to their use showed the slightest sign of possible success, a long-retired scientist with a high reputation in the sphere of Chemistry or Medicine was prompted to voice the recurring slogan in praise of the metal and to reiterate the assurance that any disparaging statements were based on nothing but imagination.

In the present case, my reply in "The Times" to a distinguished correspondent who wrote in favour of aluminium was quickly followed by his personal request, couched in the most friendly terms, for information about my work and for a reprint of my monograph. So the eminent scientist, who wrote to "The Times" in praise of aluminium kitchen utensils, had apparently not even read my monograph before writing. Perhaps it was not a very farfetched assumption that the old boy had been coaxed into putting his signature to a letter not entirely of his own writing.

Though it continued to be widely discussed in private homes, the matter was once more silenced in the press. The aluminium industry had once more got the better of Medicine. It was not that Medicine was defeated by the industry on the purely medical question as to whether aluminium kitchenware was or was not detrimental to health. Much worse! Medicine was simply taken over lock, stock and barrel on this question, without the slightest vestige of an argument, or even so much as a protest. It allowed itself to be seduced, which, in the language of big business, would, I believe, be described as turning into a junior sleeping partner.

It would, of course, be utterly wrong to assume that all the members of the medical profession allowed themselves to be made the puppets of industry. Far from it. There are, to be sure, many men and women amongst them who, in accordance with the traditional oath taken on being admitted to the sacred shrine of the art of healing, would be prepared to sacrifice everything in quest for its noblest aims. The medical profession, however, like any other calling in everyday life, has a powerful organization led by a small group of men, whose primary duty it is, in accordance with the mandate obtained, to watch over the earthly interests and rights of its members. How this duty is carried out, the rank and file are unconcerned to bother about. It is, however, one thing for the leaders of the organization to guard the material interests of its members, and quite another to lay down on purely medical matters a policy which, owing to the lack of interest displayed by the rank and file, will in due course appear to be approved by the whole profession. The organization has a number of its own journals at its disposal and the individual members of the editorial boards of these journals have the right to lay down what shall or shall not be accepted for publication. This system would be equitable enough, if what was fit to appear in the columns of each journal was decided in an unbiased manner. As it is, however, a writer submitting his work for publication in any specific journal must above all be in its good books. Should he happen to be one of those, who in their desire to preserve their independence in medical outlook remain outside the organization, he is sure to be ostracized as far as the acceptance of his medical paper is concerned.

The time had come when I began to realize that the odds were pressing too heavily against me for me to hope to overcome them single-handed. The prospects of standing up successfully against a powerful industry seemed exceedingly slight.

Chapter 5: I Join The Army

The years that followed were enough to dampen my enthusiasm to continue research. I learned to be content with what I had so far achieved, without the slightest help from outside, and, indeed, in spite of all the difficulties put in my way. What I had to tell the members of my profession about the great probability, if not certainty, that fluorine was the causative agent of the disease picture described on account of its contaminating food prepared in aluminium cooking utensils, I had already said. The problem that remained to be solved, however, was how this fact could be reconciled with my observation made on numerous occasions that in order to completely cure the disease, tap water had to be replaced by a pure and wholesome drinking water and canned food to be avoided altogether. In short, it became vitally important to investigate whether fluorine, which had been found clinically to contaminate the aluminium kitchen utensils, would also be found to contaminate the drinking water and other articles of everyday food and drink. In the circumstances prevailing at the time I doubted whether this problem could be solved satisfactorily, since at the time nothing whatsoever was known about the action of fluorine on the human body when ingested in small quantities with food and drink, and analytical methods of detecting traces of the element had not been evolved. It is no exaggeration to say that the possible significance of fluorine in Medicine was at the time completely unrecognized.

One day in 1941 it was announced to the medical community that a meeting of the Section of Comparative Medicine of the Royal Society of Medicine would be held to discuss the problem of "Fluorosis in Man and Animals". This was indeed welcome news, and there was no doubt in my mind that my work would be included in the discussion.

At the meeting the speakers reported on an outbreak of a disease amongst cattle grazing near an aluminium factory and feeding on fodder exposed to the fumes emanating from it. The cattle all perished within a short time, after suffering from symptoms mainly affecting the bones, which became soft and fractured easily. This report confirmed in all details similar findings obtained some years ago by investigators in Switzerland who, moreover, produced exactly the same disease by feeding animals on fodder exposed experimentally to hydrofluoric acid or on fodder to which a salt of this acid, namely, sodium fluoride, had been added. It thus became clear beyond any shadow of doubt that the gas emanating from the aluminium factories was hydrofluoric acid, derived from the cryolite which is one of the indispensable materials used in the manufacture of the metal. The disease produced was so typical that the appropriate name of "fluorosis" was attached to it.

This epidemic of fluorosis amongst cattle was the first one to have been observed in Great Britain. The human inhabitants of the region did not escape unscathed. Dental changes, known under the name of "mottled teeth" or "mottled enamel", occurred as a result of long-continued exposure to the fumes emanating from the aluminium factory, these changes being the first visible signs of chronic fluorine poisoning.

Of my work on aluminium and fluorine not a single word was mentioned. I sprang to my feet for this was an opportunity which I could not let slip. In the short time at my disposal I said as much as I could — that I was the first to describe a symptom-complex in man, which I frequently observed in London; that, although I had missed the changes described as occurring on the teeth, I had recorded that gingivitis and bleeding of the gums was one of the signs of the disease; and that as long as 13 years ago I had attributed it to food prepared in aluminium cooking utensils, to tap water and to canned food. I showed the sketch, taken from my monograph on aluminium, of a furnace in which bauxite and the fluorine-bearing cryolite are mixed, and I pointed out that the resulting metal was bound to contain fluorine.

To judge from the reception of what I said at this well-attended meeting, I had every reason to be pleased and to feel that my work was not entirely wasted after all, The next day I received a letter from the chairman of the meeting, asking me to send him an extract of my contribution to the discussion for inclusion in a report to be published in the Proceedings of the Royal Society of Medicine. A few days later, however, another letter came from the secretary of the Society, informing me that my manuscript had regretfully been rejected by the editors, and expressing the hope that I would accept the appreciation of the audience, which had followed my part in the discussion, as a fitting tribute.

My nature is such that obstacles in my chosen path merely increase my determination to follow it. Since my attention was at that meeting for the first time drawn to the dental changes as the first external, easily detectable sign of a systemic disease produced by the long-continued action of fluorine, mottling of the teeth became for me a matter of the utmost importance. To be sure, many of my patients whom I believed to be suffering from chronic fluorine poisoning had had gingivitis as one of its signs, but although there was a possibility that I missed the simultaneous presence of mottling of the teeth, it was more likely that mottling was absent from them. If now I could only have the opportunity of examining a sufficiently large number of people, any co-existence of "mottled teeth" with those signs and symptoms of chronic fluorine poisoning which I had already recorded would clinch the matter once and for all. The great question, however, was how to set about finding such an opportunity.

At this stage of the war, medical officers were urgently needed for services in the army. What about offering my services in spite of my being above military age? If they were accepted, I should have a unique opportunity to investigate the problem on a large scale.

My hopes materialized. I left my patients to look after themselves as best they could. So far as I myself was concerned, my life in the army for the duration of the war would differ markedly from that I had led in surroundings that had become intolerable, and I decided to make the best of the opportunity that was offered me.

The batch of medical men who joined the army with me were all young men, most of whom had just graduated. For them army life was an adventure of a type utterly different from mine. We were now all sitting on school benches in a class-room, waiting for specialized military instruction. A major started us on our new career by telling us that now that we were going to be medical officers, we would have to be 99 per cent officers and one per cent medical men. Then the fiery sergeant-major with his bristling moustache did his best to make of us the impressive soldiers the major wanted us to be. We were marched to the barrack square for the usual drill, but the poor chap could not guess that his commands "Right turn" and "Left turn" were in my mind turned into planning how to proceed in my investigation of the problem of "mottled teeth". Then there was the sergeant who instructed us how to distinguish between the various war gases by their smell. To get an idea what modern war gases can do to friend and foe alike, we had on one occasion to run as fast as we could in and out of a little brick-walled structure in which an invisible and odourless gas was liberated, in order to make us acquainted with and to give us the experience of its action during an exposure of not more than 2-3 seconds. It is now known that this modern war gas contains hydrofluoric acid.

There was yet another sergeant, an excellent fellow who instructed us in the methods of purification of drinking water derived from rivers, lakes, ponds, etc. What I learned from him would in due course be of the greatest value in my practical investigation of the problem of fluorine.

One afternoon at tea time I was honoured by our Commanding Officer in the Officer's Mess, who asked me to take a seat next to him at the top of the table. Having learned of my keen interest in the problem of drinking water, he invited his friend, another colonel of the Royal Army Medical Corps, now retired and occupying a highly responsible position on the Metropolitan Water Board, to come and have tea with him. After introduction, we two were left to discuss the subject in which we were both vitally interested. I ventured the opinion that the London drinking water was perhaps after all not that "best drinking water in the world", as the public were made to believe. I told him point blank that, as a result of my 12 years' investigation, I had come to the conclusion that the drinking water appeared to be contaminated by fluorine. "Fluorine in the drinking water? I never heard of it," came the reply. Neither the colonel, who must have felt that he had wasted a precious afternoon in coming to meet a newly-commissioned lieutenant to discuss the problem of drinking water, nor I myself could foresee that some 12 years later we would once more cross swords over the problem of fluorine, not over a cup of tea at the Officers' Mess in the shadow of Westminster, but across the Atlantic.

No doubt following a report from the fierce-looking sergeant-major, who from his observation on the barrack square had come to the correct conclusion that I was absent-minded during drill and thereby retarded the military education of the others, my training which like that of my comrade-in-arms was intended to last three weeks was prematurely cut short. Being now passed as sufficiently trained for duties in the army, I was to report as a medical officer to a home regiment in which newly enlisted recruits, both male and female, were getting their two or three months' military training before being posted.

The Training Regiment to which I found myself attached was stationed in the country at a fair distance from London, yet near enough for me to remain in touch with medical libraries. I now mainly concentrated on studying the dental lesion bearing the attractive name of "mottled teeth". Since large intakes of new recruits coming direct from civilian life arrived in the camp once every fortnight to replace those already trained, my medical duties kept me busy only for a few days following the new intake, during which I had to classify the new arrivals according to their physical condition and to give them the various inoculations. Apart from these few days and from the hour or two of the daily "sick parades", my time was entirely my own. I very soon found that this would be the ideal milieu for my work on the problem of fluorine. Here I would have a unique opportunity to examine large numbers of young men and women recruited from every possible walk of life and coming from practically all over the country for the presence of "mottled teeth" and for any co-existence of this dental lesion with those signs and symptoms which I clinically attributed to the long-continued action of fluorine. No similar opportunity would ever have been offered outside my new army life.

The first question to be answered was: What do "mottled teeth" look like? Since apparently a large amount of literature had grown, principally in this country, before the subject came to the notice of the dental and medical professions in Great Britain, it was necessary to study it in all its aspects. Information contained in numerous articles was obtained through the courtesy of the librarian and his staff of the Royal Society of Medicine. I was also particularly fortunate in having the help of a brother officer in the camp, whose knowledge of the Spanish language enabled me to complete the study of the extensive literature on the subject that had appeared in various foreign countries. His help has proved invaluable ever since.

Chapter 6: Mottled Teeth

The study of any scientific problem requires a great deal of patience and perseverance in collecting together all the available evidence gathered by previous workers. Frequently this early evidence is confusing or even contradictory in its details and it takes a long time before a clear picture emerges, definite enough to serve as a basis for further scientific investigation.

As regards "mottled teeth", it must be assumed that they have existed in some parts of the world since time immemorial and that their occurrence did not altogether escape the attention of Medicine and Dentistry, though it is doubtful whether they attracted any particular interest in either of these two professions until recently. There is no record of any medical man's interest in the subject, and if there was any early description of the dental lesion, the time was probably not ripe for following it up owing to the mysterious nature of its origin. In short there is no documentary evidence to indicate that anything was done about it up to some 50 years ago, although it is quite certain that popular opinion had long been gravely concerned about the matter.

It was only in 1901 that the problem was brought to the fore by an American naval surgeon by the name of Eager, who was attached to a cruiser anchored in the harbour of Naples, Italy. It is likely that Eager was not kept very busy as medical officer on his cruiser, and probably when his work was done he went ashore and mingled with the indigenous population of Naples. Whilst laughing and singing their famous songs, the Neapolitans showed that their teeth were very different from normal. Eager was struck by their unfamiliar appearance, and he made numerous inquiries. He learned a great deal about their teeth from the people, and as he listened to their story his curiosity grew. He was told that their teeth were spoken of as "denti di Chiaie", because a man of this name was said to have reported on them a long time age, although no documentary evidence could ever be found to that effect. Since in many cases the teeth assumed a black appearance, they were sometimes referred to as "denti neri" or as "denti scritti", when they looked as if written upon. Popular belief attributed the condition to the climate, to the vapours emanating from the Vesuvius, and even to the sins of previous generations or to the Devil himself. Some thought that they might be due to the drinking water.

True to the reputation of his progressive countrymen, Eager sat down at the desk in his cabin and wrote out a report on what he

31

had seen and what he had heard concerning the teeth of the population of Naples. The report which was published in the widely-read "Dental Cosmos" was short, to the point, and impressive. It immediately caught the imagination of the dental profession all over the country. Their attention drawn to what now became known as mottling of the teeth, dentists began to look out for any occurrence of the lesion in this country. Soon reports came in, one after another: Yes, mottled teeth were to be seen in this country as well. Discussions at numerous dental meetings followed, at which an endeavour was made to shed some light on the causation of the unsightly appearance of the victims' teeth.

It was some 15 years later, that two American dentists, Black and McKay, after a thorough study of the problem, published in 1916 a comprehensive description of the lesion from all aspects. Their findings were so accurate that to this day they form a basis for any further study of the problem.

The upper front teeth are usually affected most. In the mildest form of mottling, light brown stains appear on the surface of the teeth, their colour being very much like that of tobacco. Later there develop milk-white or paper-white specks and patches varying in size and shape, and horizontal bands of varying width. Sometimes the whole surface of the teeth loses its normal glossy translucency and assumes a dull, chalky-white appearance. As the condition progresses, pits appear on the surface of the teeth, first retaining the normal colour and later turning brown or even black. Their distribution in quite characteristic: They form a straight line running in an oblique direction across the tooth, one pit close to the other as if they were links of a chain, or they are irregularly scattered all over the surface giving it a coarse, honeycombed appearance.

The arrangement of the teeth is often very irregular. They are crowded together and grow in a disorderly fashion. Their front surface in many cases turning to the side. The cutting edge is frequently prematurely and excessively worn out. The teeth become brittle, and in advanced cases so loose that they can easily be pulled out with the fingers. Whilst the description of the physical changes of these teeth was perfect from every point of view, the cause of the lesion remained as obscure as ever. Of the various theories adduced one particularly appealed to McKay. Since a widespread popular belief maintained that the drinking water might be at fault, he suggested in 1918 that, in order to settle this question once and for all, a grandiose experiment should be carried out, not in a laboratory but in a practical manner, by replacing the drinking water in an area where "mottled teeth" were encountered with water from an area where none could be observed. As if by a miracle, the generation of children drinking the water derived from the new supply had teeth free from mottling. The older people, whose teeth were already mottled, did not benefit by the change of water supply and their teeth remained mottled.

Here was incontrovertible proof that the cause of the dental lesion was indeed contained in the drinking water. Further research was henceforth greatly facilitated since it was now possible to discard all the other theories hitherto considered and to concentrate on what was no longer theory but fact. Dental investigators, together with those from other branches of science, chiefly physiologists and biochemists, busied themselves in trying to find out precisely what was contained in the drinking water in certain areas which produced mottling of the teeth.

Research of this kind is not much talked about outside the laboratories concerned. The public gets acquainted with it only when everything is satisfactorily completed. Any failures, of which there are many on the hard path of a research worker, are simply set aside or forgotten. It was another 13 years before three American investigators, Smith, Lantz and Smith, were able in 1931 to convey the important message to the world of science that the factor contained in the drinking water which produced mottling of the teeth was found. It was fluorine, an element belonging, together with chlorine, iodine and bromine, to a chemical group called the halogens.

As little as one part of fluorine dissolved in a million parts of drinking water, or 1 mg. of the poison in a litre of drinking water, equivalent to 1/120th part of a grain in a pint of water, is sufficient to produce mottling of the teeth, when ingested during the period of calcification of the teeth, that is to say, during the first 8 years of life. When the calcification is completed at the age of 8 years, no mottling will occur as a result of subsequently drinking a water polluted by fluorine. Mottling of the teeth is thus brought about through the fluorine ingested being absorbed into the general blood circulation and damaging the teeth.

At the same time another American, Churchill, found spectroscopically that in areas in which "mottled teeth" were endemic the drinking water contained more fluorine than in areas where no mottling was observed.

Numerous investigations followed, at first confined to this country but soon in other parts of the world. The knowledge of the role which fluorine played in the causation of dental changes thus became the property of the world of natural sciences and gave an ever-increasing stimulus to a large number of investigators outside Dentistry, foremost amongst them again physiologists and biochemists, in the search for further damage which might be caused by the long-continued ingestion of fluorine. Important results were obtained, and they not only fully confirmed those obtained in animal experiments with fluorine at the end of the 19th and the beginning of the present century, but further extended the knowledge of the effects of the poison on various organs and their organic functions.

Whilst notable progress was thus being made in gradually revealing the deleterious action of fluorine, albeit only by isolated and uncoordinated studies of its effect on the teeth of man and on various organs of experimental animals, in Great Britain there was as yet little evidence of any interest being taken in the subject. This may have principally been due to the characteristic tendency of the British medical profession of waiting, to see the direction being taken by research in other countries. The apathy, however, was to cease after that meeting at the London Royal Society of Medicine. In the army camp, after making an extensive and methodical study of what had so far been achieved, I commenced an extensive, practical study of the subject.

The first vital question to solve was the incidence of "mottled teeth" in the country. Having in the course of my work gone through the hard school of experience, I knew that there were pitfalls to guard against. If I, a medical man without a specialized knowledge of dentistry, had examined the people's teeth for the presence of mottling, my findings would soon be exposed to the charge of unreliable investigation. Because of the primitive knowledge of the subject that prevailed generally it would be objected that what I looked upon as being "mottled teeth" (because of the milk-white specks, patches and horizontal lines, which were now universally accepted as being due to fluorine) should be called by other names, for example "dental hypoplasia", and ascribed to other causes, such as rickets, infectious diseases of childhood, lack of vitamins, etc. To forestall such objections, it was necessary to invite the help of a dentist familiar with the subject, I found one serving in a military camp adjacent to my own. We were fortunate in securing the collaboration and the permission of the Commanding Officer of the camp to examine the large numbers of recruits, both male and female, after the hours of their daily military training. Having been fully informed of the purpose of the investigation, the recruits voluntarily sacrificed part of their time off duty.

Small-scale examination of the teeth of school children living in isolated communities had already been carried out by other investigators, and this had shown that mottling was prevalent amongst them. The present investigation, however, was the first carried out on several thousand young men and women living in various parts of the country, and it revealed that mottling was in a variable degree widespread amongst the whole population of Great Britain. No relationship could be established between the age of those having "mottled teeth" and the degree of mottling. There were many instances of young men and women found to have mottled teeth far advanced, and older ones showing only slight lesions. It could, however, be ascertained even at this early stage of the investigation that in principle there is no difference between the action of fluorine and that of any poison, inasmuch as the extent of the harm depends above all on the quantity ingested and on the length of time during which it has been taken.

The teeth of the British population are generally reputed to be bad. The present investigation soon confirmed that this unenviable reputation was fully justified. This accounted for the fact that a large proportion of those examined were found to have been fitted with dentures to replace teeth extracted at an early age.

A final analysis of the findings obtained revealed that about every fourth person amongst the thousands examined had mottled teeth to some extent. Even this high proportion represented a conservative figure, since any doubtful and all the edentulous cases were placed in the category of those whose teeth were not mottled, although at least some of the extracted teeth were no doubt mottled in their time.

Chapter 7: Plenty Of Harm Caused By Fluorine

It has already been explained that mottling of the teeth is the result of drinking a water containing a concentration of at least 1 part per million of fluorine ingested during the first 8 years of life. Mottling of the teeth is not a localized lesion, but the first visible, external sign of chronic fluorine poisoning produced via the general blood circulation. These facts are firmly established, and no attempt will ever succeed in explaining them away. On them will henceforth rest the study of every other aspect of the problem. The fact that the incidence of the dental lesion had been found to be widespread in Great Britain could not fail to help shed considerable light on the subject.

Having been ingested with the drinking water into the alimentary canal, from which it is absorbed into the general blood circulation, the poison must necessarily be carried into every corner of the body, coming in close contact with the whole system. Even though fluorine, like any other poison, exerts a preference for one tissue or one organ over another, it is bound to some extent to affect every one of them. This means interference with their normal function, in other words, impaired health.

I had now as many as 1,099 people with mottled teeth at my disposal for further study. The next step was to try to find out whether mottling of the teeth was accompanied by any complaints of impaired health, and more especially to see whether the various signs and symptoms of the disease which for several years past, even before I knew anything of the dental lesion, I had attributed to the long-continued action of fluorine were coexistent. It must be borne in mind that these were mainly young people, who had just been recruited from civilian life for service in the army following one or more medical examinations. I could not expect, therefore, to find any apparent illness in them. If, however, they admitted having any complaints, the significance of such complaints would be gauged by the frequency of their co-existence with "mottled teeth".

The following simple questions were put to the people whose teeth were mottled:

1. *Do you take salts, pills, or any other aperients? Do you suffer from constipation?*
2. *Do you ever have "pins and needles" in your fingers? Do they go dead and numb?*
3. *Have you ever had any boils?*

4. *Do you at any time have heat-spots, heat-bumps, or rashes?*
5. *Do you ever notice loose, shrivelled skin between the toes? Does it peel?*
6. *Does your hair fall out?*
7. *Are your finger nails brittle? Do they break easily?*

Of the 1,099 cases with mottled teeth, only 125 did not complain of any of these symptoms. All the others, however, did complain of one or several of them in a variable degree. It was concluded that the co-existence of these symptoms with mottled teeth was not merely a matter of coincidence, but that they formed an integral part of the symptomatology of chronic fluorine poisoning. Thus the presence of mottled teeth represented only one, a minor aspect of the picture, whilst the other symptoms brought into view the medical side. The hitherto purely dental problem had hence become a purely medical subject which, as far as man was concerned, had till now been entirely overlooked.

Amongst the symptoms here enumerated, obstinate constipation was the one most frequently encountered. It was followed by the sensation of "pins and needles" in the fingers and hands, by boils, weals and rashes of various kinds, by loss of hair and by brittleness of the nails, in this order. Loss of hair was a distinct feature and attracted special attention when the victims were young men. In a few cases it was so pronounced that, even before the teeth were examined, chronic fluorine poisoning was suspected as being the cause of it. The examination of the teeth promptly confirmed the suspicion and, as a rule, other signs and symptoms here enumerated completed the disease picture.

In interrogating those afflicted with mottled teeth, great care was taken to select only such signs and symptoms from amongst those clinically found to be due to the action of fluorine as could not possibly be subject to any mistake or to psychological influences. Those which could be misinterpreted in any way were omitted altogether so as to avoid wrong conclusions.

The frequent co-existence of damage to the skin, teeth, nails and hair is not merely an accident, since in embryonic life the three last-named organs develop from the skin, of which they form a part. Moreover, all the four organs take their origin from what is called the ectoderm, the outer layer of a structure representing the earliest phase of the embryonic life. It is for this reason that they are called ectodermal organs. Damage to the ectodermal organs is spoken of as ectodermal lesions.

The ectodermal organs are regulated by internal glands known as parathyroids. There are four of these in number, embedded in the upper and in the lower surface of both the right and the left lobe of the thyroid. Their function is to regulate the calcium content of the body, a material as indispensable for sustaining health and life as is oxygen. If they are damaged, their function is lowered. This leads to a reduction of the normal amount of calcium stored in the body and to injury to the various ectodermal organs.

Apart from the skin and its appendages, the teeth, nails and hair, the nervous system is also derived from the ectoderm. The toxic action on the nervous system manifests itself in neuralgiae, in cramps, and in the sensation of "pins and needles", etc. — all of which I have already described as being the result of a long-continued ingestion of fluorine.

Whilst it thus becomes obvious that the skin, the teeth, the nails, the hair and the nervous system are not, each of them separately, attacked by fluorine in a direct manner but through the agency of the parathyroid glands, there is definite evidence that any injury to these glands, whether accidental or through the action of fluorine, produces a disease which is identical with the one here described. It is called tetany. It will depend on the degree of the accidental damage or on the amount of fluorine ingested whether the ensuing tetany will be acute and possibly kill the victim within a few days or even hours, or whether it will take a slow chronic course in which the victim complains of the signs and symptoms here described. Cases are known, in which a large dose of a fluorine salt has been swallowed by mistake or in attempted suicide or in homicide; acute tetany was the result, and unless immediate treatment was given before the fluorine had time to do irreparable damage, the victim died. As a main part of the treatment, calcium is given in large amounts so as to replace the calcium which fluorine had removed from the body. If, on the other hand, only small quantities of fluorine are ingested over a long period of time, chronic tetany is the result. Whereas, however, to produce mottled teeth the poison must have been ingested during the first 8 years of life, the other signs and symptoms of chronic tetany occur following the ingestion of fluorine at any age.

There is yet further evidence to the effect that mottling of the teeth is brought about through the interference of the ingested fluorine with the function of the parathyroid glands. Nearly 50 years ago, at a time when medical investigators were busy trying to determine the action of these newly discovered glands, experiments were carried out on rats consisting in the removal of these glands. This resulted in tetany, of which one important sign was dental changes in the form of white decalcified stripes across the teeth. There were also sores on the body and loss of hair, but their significance was at the time misinterpreted, inasmuch as they were thought to be the effect of mites pervading the skin. Some 25 years later, when Dentistry in this country was preoccupied with the problems of mottled teeth, those white decalcified stripes across the teeth of the experimental rats were recalled, and it was found that the lesions were in every respect similar in both cases.

It is thus clear that chronic fluorine poisoning is identical with chronic tetany. In either of them, the numerous complaints here enumerated linger for a long time without killing the victim. During his long illness, other diseases of which the cause is at present obscure, may develop. Only time and further clinical and experimental study will show whether any connexion exists between chronic fluorine poisoning, on the one hand, and those other diseases of a hitherto unknown origin, on the other.

Chapter 8: Fluorine In The Drinking Water

No time was to be wasted. The length of service of a medical officer in any army unit was unpredictable, and there was always the possibility that I might without warning be transferred to another place, where perhaps no similar facilities would be available for further work. I had to strike while the iron was hot, and to snatch at every opportunity whilst it offered.

Since fluorine present in the drinking water alone was believed to produce mottling of the teeth, my attention was now concentrated on studying the nature of the drinking water. I was anxious to learn how to carry out the medical analysis for fluorine, and fortunately I became friendly with the head of the Department of Chemistry at the renowned Faculty of Agriculture of Reading University, not far away from my camp. His help was invaluable in imparting the specialized knowledge of how the concentration of fluorine could be determined in any given sample of drinking water.

It so happened that a comparatively large number of recruits in the camp were at the time afflicted with an outbreak of boils and other skin troubles. The cause of this became clear when we ascertained that the drinking water contained as much as 1.4 parts per million of fluorine, nearly 50% above the concentration which is known to produce mottling of the teeth in children as the first visible sign of chronic fluorine poisoning, of which recurrent attacks of boils are one of many other manifestations. In addition to my own camp duties, I was at that time assigned to carry out medical duties in a highly confidential unit located near-by in the secluded private grounds and country house belonging to a brewer. The brewer seems for a long time to have had his own suspicions about the quality of the drinking water supplied to his property, so he installed his own plant, identical with one which is generally employed for the filtration and purification of water used in brewing beer.

This plant consists of a tank filled with aerated water, which is pumped into a metal container. Inside the container is housed the filter. A quantity of a white powder suspended in water is poured in, a manufactured product of a mineral which contains an aluminium compound as a basic constituent. It is mainly the absorptive power of the aluminium that is utilized in the process of water purification. The water to be purified comes into intimate contact with the powder and on leaving the filter is ready for drinking and cooking purposes

It became a matter of great interest to find out whether samples of this powder did contain any fluorine. A quantity of the filter powder was suspended in distilled water, which had first been ascertained to be free from fluorine, and was well shaken at intervals so as to make sure that it was uniformly suspended. This examination revealed the presence of appreciable amounts of fluorine. Samples of filter powder obtained from various sources, or those obtained from one source at different periods of time, were also found to be contaminated by fluorine to a larger or lesser extent. Whilst in two cases alumina, which was used for the preliminary coagulation of organic matter in the water derived from rivers, lakes, ponds, etc., prior to chlorination and filtration, contained only insignificant traces or small amounts of fluorine, the water sterilizing powder used for the subsequent chlorination contained as much as 39 parts of fluorine per million parts of the powder, and two samples of the filter powder, which were obtained from two different leading sources of supply, were loaded with the poison in concentrations of not less than 68 and 120 parts per million respectively. Obviously, at least part of these large quantities of fluorine present in the various materials employed in the process of purification must have been absorbed into the drinking water.

At this juncture it becomes necessary to point out that the amount of fluorine found in the water does not on chemical analysis correspond with the amount of the fluorine contained in the various materials mentioned above. The reason for this is not clear. One explanation has it that, upon contact of fluorine with water, ozone is evolved and hydrofluoric acid formed which, being a gas, is only partly dissolved in the water, another part remaining free and able to escape in a volatile form. Whatever the explanation, it is a fact proved over and over again that the present method of analysis employed to detect the presence of fluorine is not to be depended on even in the hands of reliable analytical chemists and public analysts. Any material, divided into two portions and examined independently by two expert analysts, will more likely than not yield widely discrepant results. It would, therefore, be entirely wrong to rely on the findings obtained, until more accurate methods of analysis are discovered.

On one occasion my attention was drawn to a hot water pipe in the camp which was so clogged by fur that for the sake of economy, it had to be disconnected. It was made of galvanized iron, 1½ inches in diameter, but the bore was patent only to the extent of 3/8 inch. Since the powder used for water filtration has been ascertained to contain fluorine, and the drinking water in the camp had a concentration of 1.4 parts per million of fluorine, the examination of the fur promised to be fruitful. Analysis showed it to contain appreciable amounts of fluorine.

The question arose whether there was any fluorine in the cement or concrete with which deep wells and many water storage tanks are built, particularly since it is known that workers handling cement are often affected by an eczema on their fingers and hands, which is identical with the eczema on the fingers and hands of people who are allergic to fluorine ingested with various articles of food and drink, of whom I was one. Analysis of samples of the materials used for mixing cement and concrete revealed that they, too, contained large amounts of fluorine as an impurity. It is not far fetched to assume that drinking water stored in cement tanks will be contaminated.

On another occasion I was ordered to inspect the water supply laid in a newly designed military camp. A main water supply with a fluorine content of 0.4 parts per million of fluorine was tapped off by means of old iron pipes, which had been recovered from some bomb-damaged houses, to feed a part of the camp. A few weeks later, this branch supply was extended to another part of the new camp by means of old iron pipes which were rusty and corroded. A sample of water drawn from the first section was estimated to contain as much as 1.4 parts per million, and that from the extension not less than 2 parts per million of fluorine. There can be no doubt that, in the present case, the increase of the fluorine content in the samples of the drinking water, drawn from taps which were placed at a distance of not more than a few hundred yards, must be attributed to the old, rusty, and corroded iron pipes. This conclusion was drawn in another locality, where water derived from a chalk containing only negligible quantities of fluorine was found to contain as much as 2.4 parts per million of fluorine after it had left the storage tank made of iron. It is now an established fact that metals are frequently contaminated by fluorine.

It occurred to me that it would be interesting to investigate how the drinking water in the camp, with its appreciable fluorine content, would respond to boiling in vessels made of different materials, such as glass, tin, enamel, aluminium and stainless steel. The fluorine content of the water, as it came out of the tap, was once more confirmed. On boiling, the water became turbid, but the degree of turbidity varied in the different vessels. On cooling, the deposit settled. The fluid on top of the deposit was then examined, and it was found that in each case boiling resulted in a considerable reduction, practically amounting to complete disappearance, of the fluorine content. The degree of reduction depended on the length of time of boiling.

This was indeed a surprising finding, in fact so surprising that, having repeated the experiment a few times, always with the same result, I decided to leave the test-tubes undisturbed to be re-examined in due course. I considered it necessary to make sure that there was no error of analysis, before jumping to any conclusions.

A still bigger surprise was to come when, on re-examining the contents of the test-tubes after a lapse of 2 or 3 days, I found that the water, which after boiling had its concentration of fluorine considerably reduced, now had it increased again, though not to the original level. There was not the slightest doubt in my mind as to the correctness of my findings obtained on both occasions.

The phenomenon seemed to me to be of great importance, but I have not seen it described before. My expert chemist friend from Reading University had to be consulted. I still vividly see him arriving in my camp on his bicycle, as well as my officer friend hurrying from his office in the camp to my room, in which I had carried out the experiment, to witness the controlled repetition of the analyses. That part which could be carried out on the spot, up to letting the boiled water cool down for a few days, was fully confirmed; that is to say, it was definitely established once and for all that if a sample of water, which showed appreciable temporary hardness, was boiled it would have the greater part of its fluorine content removed. Obviously, the fluorine must have gone somewhere in the process of boiling, and it was demonstrated with the greatest of ease that it was now present in the solid deposit of calcium carbonate, which as a result of boiling came down to the bottom of the vessel. My chemist friend took with him to his laboratory an ample supply of the original drinking water, so as to repeat the experiment once more to examine the boiled water after the deposit had been left undisturbed for a few days. This finding was also confirmed.

All these findings revealed a new, hitherto unknown, characteristic of hard drinking water containing fluorine. They may not apply to the same extent if the water so treated is soft, as pointed out by investigators in London who duplicated the experiment, even though in their case also the fluorine content was slightly reduced. It was, however, a few years later that a report appeared in the Bulletin of the noted Swiss Academy of Medical Sciences to the effect that a method had been discovered by which fluorine contained in food and drink could be removed. That method was boiling. To be sure, its author came to this conclusion independently, without knowing that the whole of my experiment had already been reported under the signature of my chemist friend and myself as far back as 1943. It was, for this reason, all the more encouraging to learn that the important finding had been fully confirmed, albeit only in so far as it concerned the first part of the experiment, namely, the effect on the fluorine in the water immediately after boiling. Unfortunately, the Swiss investigator did not carry out the second part of the experiment, showing the effect of re-solution of the deposit after prolonged cooling.

The process of transferring the fluorine present in the hard water into the deposit of calcium carbonate by means of boiling appears to be mechanical rather than chemical. To it is probably due the finding prescribed above, which showed fluorine to be present in the fur removed from the hot water pipe. To keep the boiled drinking water free from fluorine, it would be necessary to decant it immediately after boiling, so as to separate it from the deposit carrying the fluorine, before the deposit had time to redissolve once more.

As a result of the experiments here described, the various unfounded theories about the mysterious, hitherto inexplicable origin of the fluorine in the water will have to be discarded once and for all. There can be no doubt that the fluorine content in the water is not necessarily always derived from the soil in the way that it has hitherto been believed to be derived, namely, through the water coming in contact with the soil and minerals containing fluorine in its course from its origin down to the well. The presence in the water of toxic amounts of fluorine is not always an act of God, but often one of civilized man.

Chapter 9: I Receive A Raspberry

My work in the camp depended to a large extent on the goodwill of the officers commanding the various companies. Their help and collaboration was well-nigh indispensable. Not all of them, however, were able to appreciate the magnitude of the problem. The explanation that mottling of the teeth was only of secondary importance in the disease picture of chronic fluorine poisoning, in which much more serious issues were at stake, was quite beyond the comprehension of some of them. A few were definitely hostile to what they thought was an undesirable interference with the routine activities of army life.

Many months of hard work went by, taking up every available hour of my spare time. Findings obtained from the examinations of thousands of men and women for signs and symptoms of chronic fluorine poisoning and from the investigation of the various aspects of the nature of the drinking water had to be correlated with the results of all the work that had ever been published on subjects which might have any bearing on the problem. The material obtained from studying this extensive literature and the evaluation of the results of my own work had to be written out in the form of articles for publication in medical journals. This was a time-absorbing task, as important as the investigation itself, but at any rate it was not affected by my surroundings. Sitting in my room at a desk piled with dozens of books, papers, reports, etc., I would write, alter, re-write, and improve on the text and form of presentation of the articles. Deeply engrossed in my work, I would often have to be reminded at a late hour that dinner was finished and that I would have to hurry up if I wanted to get some food.

This mode of life did not by any means harmonize with the mode of life of many of my brother-officers. For them, quite legitimately, work was finished at a certain hour of the day. After dinner, they would form a party of a dozen or so and pay their daily visit to the village pub, where "lifting the elbow" would help to relax their overworked minds. This habit became part of their routine life, although it did not necessarily appeal to every one of them. It certainly did not appeal to me, owing to my allergy to the fluorine content of the beer. I preferred to stay in my room reading and writing, often up to a late hour of the night. In fact, the blissful quiet in the camp late in the evening was the most fruitful time for me to complete my articles on the various aspects of my subject. I felt I had no time for leisure and social conviviality, although I knew well enough that isolating oneself from the others after the hours of duty was not encouraged in army life.

Clouds started to gather on the horizon, and signs of suspicion became evident. Gradually a whispering campaign against my work began to be carried on. The question: "What is the real object of all this business?" was raised on a few occasions. It was remarked that it was unusual for a medical officer to remain attached to one unit for as long as I was. I felt instinctively that the time was fast approaching when I should be posted away to another unit.

There was one more bit of research to be carried out in the camp, if possible. Since the fluorine concentration of our drinking water was known to me to be 1.4 parts per million, it would be profitable to trace the water supply back to its origin and to find out whether there was any variance in the fluorine content. True, this would be repetition of work which I had already done on a water supply outside the camp, but it was my desire to bring home to the higher military authorities that it would be in the interest of the troops to check my findings and to rectify matters, if necessary. I knew by now that the procedure to be adopted was to approach my immediate superior medical officer in the area, and to ask his permission "to examine the source of the water supply a few miles away from the camp. When I told him of my plans, he looked at me as if I were not in my right senses. He was, of course, cognizant of the rumours in my camp, and he felt that my activities were not compatible with the duties of a medical officer in the army. He remarked significantly that I appeared to have too much time on my hands at my present post. No, I would not have his permission to carry out the proposed examination. Pleading that my investigation did no harm to anybody and that my purely medical duties were not interfered with was of no avail. In army slang, I had been given a raspberry. I quickly recovered my composure, however, for after all what was a raspberry, the first raspberry in my military career, or a hundred raspberries for that matter, in comparison with my desire to continue my work on fluorine.

Having left the presence of my senior medical officer by the front door, I decided to approach my problem by the back entrance. My medical duties, I tried to persuade myself, had nothing to do with my investigation of the problem of fluorine. I, therefore, decided to invite the help of the garrison adjutant, who had military jurisdiction over the water supply in the area. He in turn sent me to the civilian Commissioner of the Water Works, and promised also to obtain further information for me. I explained to the civilian Commissioner of the Water Works the nature of my work, and without even as much as mentioning the lack of cooperation on the part of my senior medical officer, I asked him to help me examine a sample of the drinking water supplied direct from the source. He seemed quite agreeable, showed me on a map the various sources from which the water was drawn before undergoing the process of purification, and promised to give me an appointment by letter in a day or two to inspect the place together with him.

After a day or two, however, a letter arrived marked to be handed to me personally against my signature. It read as follows:

CONFIDENTIAL
Subject: Enquiries regarding water supply.
Lieutenant .L. Spira, R.A.M.C.
M.O. i/c Troops

Reference attached copy of letter to you. I understand that you are now making private enquiries concerning the source, etc. of local water supplies. As under present conditions such enquiries by you are likely to arouse considerable suspicion as to your reason or authority for making such investigation, I write to give you orders that all such enquiries whether private or official will be discontinued forthwith.
(Sig.) •••••• Lieut-Colonel
Copy to: Garrison Adjutant

The attached copy mentioned in that letter read as follows:

Subject: Water Supply
To: Lt. Spira, R.A.M.C.

Reference your request for information concerning the water supply system and the sources from which the water is derived.
I regret that I am unable to obtain this information for you as your enquiries are not of an official nature.
(Sig.) • • • • • • • • • Major
Garrison Adjutant

During the war, however "confidential" letters of this kind might be, their contents were bound to become known and offer a welcome distraction from the numerous monotonous daily rumours. Here at last was something to warm one's heart! Rumours quickly spread all over the camp. The medical officer had at last been caught out! An enemy agent, he had tried to obtain access to the public water supply and to poison it with arsenic, not in a local reservoir but at the source itself!

It looked as if things were going to get lively. Obviously, the next step would be a court martial. After many months of anxiety there would be an acquittal, and after the acquittal, I decided, I would abandon the King's uniform. After all, whatever was in store for me, I had achieved during my short military career practically everything I set out to achieve, and the foundation for further work on the problem of fluorine had been laid, for others, if not for myself.

There was not the slightest bitterness in my heart. Instead, there was a feeling of sincere gratitude for the great opportunity I had had of achieving important results by hard work, an opportunity which did not spontaneously come my way but one which I took, as one takes the bull by the horns. It would be idle to deny that my gratitude was mixed with feelings of pessimism about human nature. But will human nature ever change?

During the weeks that followed I waited, expecting a case to be made out against me by higher quarters. Apart from the little "sick parade" in the medical inspection room every morning, my time was spent working continuously on articles, which were in due course to record my findings in medical journals.

Chapter 10: The General Pays A Visit

During the war army regulations required anything intended for publication to be submitted for approval to the War Office in London. The material would have to go through a strict censorship at various levels of the army hierarchy, starting with the office of the senior medical officer in the area. After several weeks of close scrutiny to find out whether the material submitted contained anything that might be useful to the enemy, it would come back along the same ladder, from London down to the office of the senior medical officer. Having passed the censorship, permission would be given to have the paper published in a medical journal.

Several of my manuscripts were sent in quick succession to the War Office for approval. Sometimes a new manuscript was on the way to London, before the previous one was returned with the permission to have it published. No exception appears to have been taken against any one of them. On the contrary. On one occasion, I was rung up from London and asked whether, in view of the long time I would have to wait to have my paper published in one of the leading medical journals, I would not like to have it immediately accepted for publication in the official organ of the Royal Army Medical Corps. The request came too late: the paper had already been accepted by a leading medical journal, subject to its being passed by the censors. Whilst the attention of the medical authorities at the War Office was thus occupied with my work, another of its branches must have been kept busy inquiring into the rumours concerning my activities in the camp. This looked very much like another case of Dr. Jekyll and Mr. Hyde.

One Saturday morning I was informed by the senior medical officer that an inspection would take place at my Medical Inspection Room that same afternoon soon after lunch. This sounded very unusual, for Saturday afternoon was part of the week-end for everybody in training regiments in the army, except for the few who were on duty.

One of my orderlies stood outside the little room on the lookout for the arrival of the commission to be announced. Presently four or five Rolls Royces arrived unloading some ten high ranking officers who were led by none less but the Director of the Medical Services of the district, the Lieutenant-General of the Royal Army Medical Corps himself: I have never seen a medical general and so many colonels assembled in a place as humble as mine. I was then asked to show all the books containing the entries of the sick at the daily "sick parades", etc., and to explain how in general the Medical Inspection Room was run by me.

It was my impression that the general was not displeased with what I showed and told him. After about 20 minutes of inspection the members of the commission prepared to leave. The chauffeurs started the engines of their cars, and there seemed no end to my clicking my heels and saluting in turn each of my superior officers on parting. Before entering his car, the general stopped to put one more question to me: whether I was satisfied with the food the troops were getting in the camp. "Yes, sir, I am very impressed with both the quantity and the quality of the rations." "What about the drink?" "Sir, I should not like, if I may, to discuss this matter. It is a sore point with me, and I have reported it on several occasions. I wish only to say again that I am not satisfied with the drinking water in the camp, which I found to contain toxic amounts of a highly potent poison. The name of the poison is fluorine."

What followed sounded to me like a well-rehearsed dramatic performance. Yet everything was spontaneous. Before the general had time to say anything in reply to what I reported, the major on duty in the camp, who waited on the commission on behalf of the Commanding Officer during his absence on week-end leave, stepped smartly forward and reported to the general: "Sir, I am ordered by the Commanding Officer to say that he would be most sorry to lose the services of our medical officer for whatever reason." Conveyed in my presence in a strictly military manner, the message was no less surprising to me than it was to the general. It did not help the Assistant Deputy of the Medical Services, the colonel superior in rank to my senior medical officer and a member of the inspecting commission, to object that my investigation looked to him like nothing but a hobby. The general ignored that remark and turned in the direction of another colonel of his suite, asking him to make a note of what was just reported to him. He took one more look at me, shook hands and said: "Doctor, carry on with your work, and I hope that one day something interesting will come out of this camp." These words are still ringing in my ears to the present day.

After the unbearable suspense of the last few weeks arising out of the rumours spread in the camp, I now felt completely stunned. Was this real, or what was it? And what had my Commanding Officer in mind when he sent his message to the general that he would not like to lose my services "for whatever reason"? There could be only one of two reasons: either transfer to another unit to stop the rumours circulating in the camp, or promotion to a higher rank which would also necessitate a transfer owing to its incompatibility with the simple medical duties in the present camp. I would not have liked either of these two developments to occur. I would feel happy to continue my work in the present camp in peace, and to let things take care of themselves. Yet the final words of the general were encouraging, and I decided not to give another thought to what the next step would be concerning my immediate future. I returned to my room to continue the work on the manuscript of another of my reports for publication in a medical journal.

Chapter 11: Ectodermal Lesions

My peace of mind had been quickly restored, and I felt I could now settle down to making further plans based on the assumption that, at any rate for the time being, I would be allowed to stay on in my camp undisturbed after all. There was first the necessity of bringing up to date a few reports on work already completed to be submitted for publication.

The examination of the camp's drinking water had lost much of its attraction during the long interval, especially because it would have involved the necessity of approaching the civilian Commissioner of the Water Works in the area for help once more. Moreover, what in the first instance I wanted to achieve, I had achieved, namely, drawing the attention of the highest medical authorities in the army to the existence of the fluorine problem.

Instead, a new survey suggested itself, consisting in determining the frequency with which each of the various ectodermal lesions would be encountered. This would bring the findings obtained into line with the already established incidence of "mottled teeth". It will be remembered that the significance of the co-existence of "mottled teeth" with lesions of the skin, nails, and hair was realized only after the first survey was completed. It indicated that all the ectodermal organs might be frequently affected at the same time. Whereas in the first survey the occurrence of the ectodermal lesions was investigated only in those, who had their teeth mottled, now the possibility had to be considered that the onset of the other ectodermal lesions might not be limited to the ingestion of fluorine within a certain age, as was mottling of the teeth, but could occur independently, as a result of long-continued ingestion of fluorine at any time in life. In fact, some of the changes observed on the nails were in appearance so much like those seen on the teeth that I suggested that, in analogy with the term "mottled teeth", the corresponding changes on the nails be designated simply as "mottled nails". It was thus possible that any person who was ingesting toxic amounts of fluorine, not during the first eight years but at some subsequent stage of life, would have no mottling of the teeth, but would have some of the other ectodermal lesions. Included in the new survey would be a repetition of estimating the incidence of "mottled teeth" in another large series of recruits in the camp, both male and female.

I have already pointed out that in the first survey of the incidence of "mottled teeth" great care was exercised to avoid the alleged risk of identifying mottling of the teeth due to the action of fluorine with closely similar dental changes observed in certain other systemic diseases, for example, rickets. Since then, however, I was able to arrive at a conclusion that the dental lesion in chronic fluorine poisoning is brought about via the disturbed function of the parathyroid glands. The fact that rickets, too, is produced by a deficient function of these glands rendered the previous differentiation obsolete.

In short, the purpose of the new survey was to ascertain how many people amongst those to be examined had mottling of the teeth, mottling of the nails in its various manifestations, loss of hair, or skin diseases, at any time, no account being taken of whether these lesions were or were not co-existent.

The result of this work revealed that as many as 48% of those examined exhibited some degree of mottling of their teeth. Even with this more accurate analysis, the incidence of the dental lesion did not fully reveal the true picture since, just as in the first survey, there still remained a number of people who had lost their teeth and could not be classified. The frequent occurrence of gingivitis, severe enough to cause bleeding of the gums, which was recorded even before fluorine was suspected as being the causative factor, was now fully confirmed. Malalignment of the teeth, due to crowding, with the resulting impaction, tilting and rotation of their axis was again observed. Various theories submitted in the past concerning the cause of this malposition of the teeth have never been substantiated, but in at least some cases the malposition has been attributed to endocrine disturbances.

Although mottling of the teeth is generally regarded as unfailing evidence of the ingestion of toxic amounts of fluorine in early childhood, the practically universal occurrence of mottling of the nails, as ascertained in the present survey, must be taken as a more delicate external, visible sign of their owner's long continued ingestion of fluorine. In other words, fluorine affects the nails with greater ease than it affects the teeth. In an endemic area, such as practically the whole of Great Britain has been found to be to a variable extent, a glance at the nails alone is, therefore, quite sufficient to state whether the person inspected has or has not escaped the action of fluorine.

The list of the various manifestations of "mottled nails" was headed by longitudinal striation affecting the finger-nails as often as the toe-nails. As many as 98% of the people examined were affected. Striation was always accompanied by thickened elevations alternating with shallow depressions across the nails, giving them a furrowed, wavy appearance. The toe-nails, particularly on the big toes, showed a tendency to grow sideways. Next in frequency were dull, opaque, chalky-white specks, patches or transverse lines, which were already mentioned on a previous occasion. They occurred on the surface of the finger-nails, but only rarely on the toe-nails. Pits, closely similar to those on "mottled teeth", were frequently observed, and in many cases an exaggerated transverse curvature of the toe-nails, with the nails thickened and a greyish corneous material filling the space under them.

Mottling of the nails may occur at any time in life, even at the age of two or three years, long before the teeth become mottled. Whilst there, it indicates that the victim is actually ingesting toxic amounts of fluorine. As the nails grow, the lesion grows with them towards their free edge. When clipped, they assume a normal appearance and no new lesions develop as long as the ingestion of fluorine ceases. By contrast, the marks seen on mottled teeth are permanent.

For a middle-aged man to start to lose his hair to an extent which indicates approaching baldness has from time immemorial been considered to be a "natural" process to which nobody would give a thought. When, however, loss of hair affects young men, it assumes a pathological significance, but so far no great importance has been attached to it. It is only when loss of hair is found to accompany other conditions, already known to be due to endocrine disturbances, that loss of hair, too, is suspected as being caused in the same way.

In the present survey, as many as 25% of the young men and women examined complained of their hair falling out. Amongst them a few young men were completely bald, and a great number of the victims showed the beginnings of sparseness of the hair, such as would appear to be "natural" if they were about 20 years older. In some cases loss of hair was found to be associated with brittleness and fragility of those hairs which still remained. This created the impression on the mind of the victim that his hair was growing only very slowly.

As in the case of loss of hair, so also in the case of various skin diseases the idea is gradually gaining recognition that, being frequently accompanied by other ectodermal lesions, many of them are caused not by a local factor but by endocrine disturbances. This belief is borne out by the fact that, whereas local treatment may in these cases be totally ineffective, treatment applied from within the body is often crowned by a strikingly prompt success.

There is, of course, nothing particularly novel in this modern conception concerning the mechanism through which skin diseases develop. The dermatological dogma that they represent a disturbance of the skin only, which like any other organ is liable to be affected without any reference to the rest of the body, has since time immemorial been strongly opposed by those who looked upon the skin as one link in the complicated make-up of the body. To be sure, even the most dogmatic interpretation of what is happening in the development of a skin disease takes full cognizance of the fact that the ingestion of certain chemical and other substances is capable of doing damage to the skin. A study of the extensive dermatological literature on the subject revealed that several skin diseases of a hitherto obscure origin were already attributed to a deficiency of the parathyroid glands. The agent which was primarily responsible for causing the deficiency had succeeded, however, in escaping attention.

In the present survey, certain skin diseases, which in an earlier stage of my work I was able to trace back to the action of fluorine via the parathyroid glands, were encountered very frequently. Not fewer than half of the persons examined were found to be afflicted by "athlete's foot", and 31% complained of outbreaks of boils and of weals at one time or another. The large number of people who had warts was striking. As many as 17% had them actually on their hands and fingers when inspected, but there were many more who stated that they had had warts in the past, but had had them removed. In the course of the examination, quite a number of people were found who had freckles on their skin. According to one report, a suggestion was made that there might be a correlation between "mottled teeth" and freckles which are popularly called "mottling of the skin." Others found that "mottled teeth" were pronounced in children predisposed to freckling. In 23% of the people examined small, soft-rounded, penulous appendages of the skin were observed in various parts of the body, particularly on the neck and in the armpits.

Chapter 12: Brown Pigmentation Of The Skin And The Man Without Sweat Glands

It was only when the present survey was nearing completion that I was struck by the frequent occurrence on the skin of the people examined of patches which, whilst being identical in colour with that of freckles, were much larger and were also often co-existent with ectodermal lesions. They were found on any part of the body, either singly or two, or rarely more in number and were of the light brown or dark brown colour comparable to that produced by the addition of milk to coffee. The discoloration was an obvious indication that the pigmentation of the skin was disturbed.

Pigmentation is regulated by the set of endocrine glands, amongst which the adrenals occupy a prominent position. The adrenal glands are two in number, one on top of each kidney, and are likewise of ectodermal origin. Dermatology is well acquainted with the frequent occurrence of patches of brown skin amongst the population of Great Britain, but although these patches are one of several manifestations of chronic arsenical poisoning, arsenic has never been detected in the material collected from the people afflicted. In the absence of a better explanation and for the sake of convenience, Dermatology has, therefore, agreed to retain for them the name of "birth marks" by which they are popularly known, although they have nothing in common with birth marks properly so called.

The observation of these brown patches of skin occurring in frequent coexistence with ectodermal lesions seemed to be of paramount importance in any further study of the problem of chronic fluorine poisoning. I therefore decided to organize yet another, the third, survey of as large a number of recruits as possible with a view to ascertaining their exact incidence. The work proceeded smoothly, now that it was carried out with the tacit approval of the higher military authorities. My senior medical officer still thought that he had better shut his eyes, so as not to be involved in case any difficulties ever arose in connexion with my work. However, I easily managed to obtain the permission of the officers commanding other camps in the vicinity of my own to examine the troops under their command. It was my aim to inspect a sufficiently large number of recruits to enable me to arrive at valid conclusions concerning a subject hitherto totally neglected. I felt that the results obtained would be welcomed by the medical profession who could not possibly try to explain away the existence of the brown patches of skin by attributing them to imagination and to psychological effects. They were there for anybody interested to see and verify. The result of my investigation would have to be accepted as recorded.

As many as 9.8%, that is to say, a tenth of the 4,818 people examined, were found to be afflicted. This was indeed a high incidence, and as in the case of the large number of people who in the previous survey were found to have freckles, this disturbance of pigmentation had to be looked upon as yet another external, visible manifestation of chronic fluorine poisoning the one highest order.

For me it was not enough to establish a new fact, important though it was, in the study of the subject. The logical sequence was to review certain diseases in which disturbance of pigmentation represents a prominent manifestation.

A serious illness first came to mind in which increased pigmentation is one of the leading features. In it the adrenal glands are often severely affected and, although in other cases no pathological changes can be detected, the illness is generally attributed to a disturbance in their function.

There is another disease in which disturbance of the adrenal glands manifests itself in patches of brown skin closely similar to those encountered in chronic fluorine poisoning. In it the brown patches are frequently accompanied by small pendulous appendages of skin, which are indistinguishable from those already mentioned as occurring mainly on the neck and in the armpits in people suffering from chronic fluorine poisoning.

In both these diseases, in addition to the adrenals, other endocrine glands, foremost amongst them the parathyroids, are involved, as is evidenced by the frequent co-existence with ectodermal lesions.

There is the disease picture of chronic arsenical poisoning already referred to. Comparison of its signs and symptoms with those mentioned as having been observed amongst patients suffering from an illness that at the time was of obscure origin revealed that they were closely similar. In fact, arsenic was suspected before fluorine was thought of as a factor producing illness when ingested with food and drink in everyday life.

The continued research on the problem of fluorine, as far as the observation of large numbers of apparently healthy young recruits was concerned, had now reached such a point that I did not mind when I was posted to another unit. My new surroundings did not vary to any great extent from those in which I had lived for the past 18 months. I still had much spare time on my hands, and I was able to make good use of it in connexion with my investigation.

There was now no more need to carry out further surveys, since I thought I had already observed all that was to be seen. Instead, I embarked upon the extensive reading of the works published on the hitherto insufficiently understood or often misinterpreted occurrence of ectodermal lesions, of brown patches of skin, of endocrine disturbances and of the various manifestations of tetany, and this reading helped considerably to increase the knowledge acquired in the course of my work. Amongst my observations there were some which at the time I was unable to correlate with those attributed to the long-continued ingestion of toxic amounts of fluorine. When I succeeded, however, in establishing clinically the fact that the parathyroids and the adrenals were involved, those observations took on an important significance. They concerned the frequent co-existence of enlarged breasts and of a feminine distribution of the pubic hair amongst men, giving rise to their designation of "feminized males", and indicating that yet other endocrine glands may be affected in chronic fluorine poisoning.

In studying numerous works on the subject of ectodermal defects, I came across statements made by several investigators to the effect that these defects were frequently accompanied by an abnormal appearance of the ears. Instead of being placed straight back and looking only slightly forward, the ear lobes are in these cases projected in an oblique direction at an unusual angle, constituting what is popularly known as "lop ear". Changes in the ear lobules, too, are often encountered. They are frequently attached to the sides of the face, and in pronounced cases are missing altogether.

Other investigators reported that absence of the ear lobules was often co-existent with disturbances of the endocrine glands. Taking these reports in conjunction with the findings obtained in my own work concerning the deleterious effect of the long-continued ingestion of toxic amounts of fluorine on the endocrine glands, the circle was thus completed and the veil surrounding the cause of certain congenital abnormalities of a hitherto obscure origin was lifted.

In the case of the absence of ear lobules, it must be assumed that fluorine ingested by the pregnant mother is acting on the foetus via the blood circulation, producing this unsightly appearance as one of the "stigmata of degeneration". In my own investigation as many as 36% of the people examined were found to be afflicted by an absence of the ear lobules.

Reports by various investigators were also encountered describing the co-existence of ectodermal lesions with yet another "stigmata of degeneration", such as stammer, ambidextrousness, left-handedness and biting of the finger nails. In my own survey these stigmata were found in a moderate number of people, but two other conditions, also reported as being frequently associated with ectodermal lesions, were met with quite often. As many as nearly 20% of those examined were afflicted with defective vision, astigmatism, short-sightedness and squint, and amongst the large number of women interrogated, nearly 12% complained of severe cramps during menstruation.

The atmosphere in the new camp turned out to be quite conducive to continued work on the subject of fluorine. My purely medical duties consisted mainly in checking the fitness of those personnel who were to be sent for service in the Far East, as well as in sorting out those who for reasons of health were repatriated from service overseas.

In the course of my study of the vast literature on the subject of ectodermal lesions, I often came across a description of cases in which ectodermal defects were very pronounced and others in which their presence constituted a grave problem of health. These latter cases attracted my attention all the more as only some 60 of the kind had so far been reported from all over the world. The defects concern inability to perspire owing to congenital absence of sweat glands in the skin, congenital total or partial absence of teeth, and congenital lack of hair sometimes amounting to complete baldness. The victims may lead a normal life when the weather is cool, but suffer seriously during the hot summer months or when doing hard physical work, owing to the fact that their body temperature is not regulated and kept at a normal level by means of sweating. They spend the hot parts of the day in a cellar, or they carry a bucket of cold water with them to sponge their skin and keep it damp. In hot weather their body temperature rises considerably, and they are quite incapable of performing any sort of physical labour. The cause of this rare condition was obscure, although it had been suggested by a few investigators that it might be due to endocrine disturbances. Owing to the rarity of the condition, I could not hope that I would ever have an opportunity of observing a case. As chance would have it, however, a thrilling experience was in store for me. Among the large number of soldiers to be interviewed daily, there was one who stated that he had been repatriated because of his having no sweat glands. I could not trust my own ears until he repeated his statement: "I have no sweat glands, sir!" As soon as I had realized my good fortune, I immediately set to work to investigate the case. It was an opportunity not to be missed, if the hope was to be fulfilled that as a result of thorough examination new findings might shed further light on this rare condition.

The condition proved to be a typical one from every point of view. Microscopical examination revealed complete absence of sweat glands in every part of the body; he had at no time in life had more than three teeth, all in the upper jaw; and his hair had always been as sparse as is the hair of a man of advanced age. Certain coexistent changes in the skin and nails, belonging to the same group of ectodermal lesions, as well as the presence of a large patch of brown skin, left no room for doubt that the parathyroids and the adrenals were involved in the same manner, but in a more advanced degree, as they were always found to be in chronic fluorine poisoning. His ear lobules were missing, and together with the complete absence of sweat glands this fact indicated that the development of certain organs had been retarded or altogether arrested in the course of his embryonic life by the action of fluorine in his pregnant mother, through the blood circulation.

The investigation took a long time to complete, and it was necessary to carry out numerous complicated examinations. In view of the probability that they would be fraught with many difficulties and with personal sacrifices on the part of the victim, I considered it my duty to keep him fully informed and to explain to him every step that might be necessary to bring the inquiry to a satisfactory conclusion. I wish to put on record that he unhesitatingly consented to any examination that would help to throw more light on his condition and that, in due course, might benefit victims similarly affected.

Chapter 13: The Brown Girl

The observation that the brown patches of skin were often accompanied by ectodermal lesions continued to command my utmost attention. Once this fact was established, and it had been ascertained that this disturbance of pigmentation had nothing to do with chronic arsenical poisoning in which brown patches of skin also very frequently occur, their presence assumed a significance far beyond my initial expectation. Henceforth, Medicine could not, so I thought, afford to continue to refuse to evaluate correctly the great diagnostic value of its occurrence.

Two more years passed, however, but none of the weekly medical journals which claim to provide information of the latest developments in the medical field took any notice of what I had recorded. Was the refusal to accept the significance of the brown patches of skin a matter of reluctance to admit failure, or was it the old insistence on having any new medical achievement proved beyond the slightest shadow of doubt?

It must be realized that it would be utterly impossible within a short spell of time, that is to say, within a predictable number of years — or indeed experimentally in any circumstances — to reproduce in man the brown patches of skin by the unthinkable method of adding toxic doses of fluorine to food and drink. Moreover, it would be entirely a matter of chance whether in any given case it would be just the adrenal glands which would be affected by the long-continued experimental administration of fluorine to any human being, so as to disturb their pigment regulating function. I have already pointed out that, for some not yet known reason, fluorine does not act uniformly on the entire nervous system but attacks sometimes the fibres supplying one endocrine gland and sometimes those supplying another.

Another recognized method of proving the correctness of the clinical finding that in these cases the disturbance of pigmentation in man was, in fact, caused by long-continued ingestion of toxic amounts of fluorine would, therefore, have to be applied, The method consists on cutting off every further intake of fluorine and in removing the amount of the poison accumulated in the body over a number of years, being in effect an essential part of a treatment directed against chronic fluorine poisoning. If, when this experiment was carried out the brown patches of skin disappeared, medical science would probably accept this result as a valid proof of the correctness of the clinical claims advanced. This method is known in Medicine as a "therapeutic test".

In my desire to gather as much evidence as possible in support of the findings obtained, I had to employ what in slang is known as "wangling". I did some wangling to obtain permission to have an American jeep (though not quite the latest model) put at my disposal whenever I wanted to visit several distant camps to examine more troops for signs of chronic fluorine poisoning, and more especially for the presence of brown patches of skin,

In the meantime, I was once again transferred to another camp in which one day my attention was drawn to the case of a woman-sergeant, who might, it was thought, interest me on account of a strange discoloration of her face. I was told that the sergeant had recently turned into a negress. She gave the following history:

Her grandfather was a negro from West Nigeria, who married a white English woman. The issue of the marriage was a son born in England, the father of the sergeant. Her father, a half-caste, was not black but very dark brown. He, too, married a white English woman. Besides her, there were two sisters and one brother, all quadroons born in England and residents in it since birth. Their skin was pale cream in colour.

Up to the age of 42, the colour of her whole body was cream, exactly like that of her brother and sisters, except that a few years ago, she noticed a brown patch on her abdomen. At the age of 42, however, a change occurred in her face, slight at first but getting gradually worse. She was always fond of sunlight, though very susceptible to it. When exposed to the sun, the skin became red and irritated. There was scaling in a scurf-like manner, leaving as time went on, a brown discoloration of an ever increasing intensity. After each attack of peeling and flaking, the face turned gradually darker, until the present permanent deep colour was reached.

When I examined her, the pigmentary changes had affected the skin of her face, giving her a grotesque appearance. The pigmentation consisted of several small patches of colour ranging from a light or dark brown to a slaty-black. There was no sharp demarcation between these patches, which merged imperceptibly into each other. The neck was also pigmented, but much less than the face. The skin of the rest of the body was of a uniformly pale-cream colour, comparable to the slightly sunburned skin of a white woman. On the cream-coloured ground, two large brown patches were present, identical with those seen frequently among the white population of Great Britain, as well as numerous "freckles" on various parts of the body. Some of the ectodermal lesions were co-existent.

She had been seen recently by various medical men, including dermatologists, all of whom arrived at the conclusion that her facial pigmentation was racial in origin. Her condition was considered to be one of those rare cases of "atavistic pigmentation", a pigmentation which, having been characteristic of many previous generations, has for some reason skipped one or more of them but has subsequently reverted to the original type.

The co-existence of the two large brown patches and of the numerous "freckles" on the normal-looking skin, as well as of some of the ectodermal lesions, all of which I attributed to the long-continued action of toxic amounts of fluorine, threw considerable doubt in my mind on the conception of "atavistic pigmentation" in this case. Instead, I remembered that during the famine years of World War I in Vienna, Austria, many cases of a similar facial pigmentation were encountered, and they were attributed to some kind of poison which adulterated the ersatz food and was by necessity ingested by the population at that time. The nature of the poison has never been ascertained, and the disease, which subsequently was observed in many other countries all over the world, even where there was no famine, remained as obscure as ever.

The facial pigmentation of the "brown girl", by which name she now became generally known, was in my opinion identical with that first recorded in Vienna, and may well have been caused by the action of fluorine ingested with various articles of food and drink, which made the skin sensitive to sunlight. An extensive investigation followed, and as it advanced it indicated that the function of the adrenal glands was disturbed.

So that a few more tests might be carried out, the patient was admitted to the hospital for what was thought would be only a few days. Whilst there, however, she became ill with severe rheumatic pains in various parts of the body. Every conceivable treatment failed to produce any improvement, and she was confined to bed, crippled for nine months, totally unable to move.

At this point, I suggested treatment directed against chronic fluorine poisoning, so as to see whether the facial discoloration if not the severe rheumatism, would thereby be influenced in any way. This treatment, carried out under the strict supervision of the medical and nursing staff of the hospital over a period of four months, resulted in a practically complete disappearance of the pigmentation. The patient could now easily pass for a woman whose face was sunburnt. The two brown patches of skin on her body likewise disappeared. Microscopical examination of the skin over the formerly slaty-black areas confirmed that, in comparison with the examination carried out before treatment, the pigment had for all practical purposes vanished. The rheumatism began to improve at the same time as the discoloration on the face showed the first signs of disappearance. A few months later our sergeant was on her feet again, fit and happy as she was before the onset of discoloration some six years previously. The "therapeutic test" proved that the severe pigmentation was indeed caused by nothing but the long-continued ingestion of toxic amounts of fluorine in this highly allergic person.

At the time of writing these lines, seven years after the first, and four years after the second report on this case appeared in one of the world's leading dermatological journals in Stockholm, Sweden, so far as I am aware, none of the British or American weekly medical journals have taken any interest in the medical aspect of the pigmentation caused by fluorine. It looks as if the mere mention of fluorine as a purely medical problem continues to be taboo.

Chapter 14: My Desperate Endeavours To Obtain Facilities To Carry Out Animal Experiments

It was quite conceivable that the more sceptical section of the medical profession would reject evidence supplied by the "therapeutic test". The "therapeutic test", they would argue, means nothing, since any improvement in the patient's condition may have been but a coincidence, a "remission", a temporary rally occurring in the course of any illness. "Post hoc", they would learnedly say, does not mean "propter hoc"; an improvement or even a cure, following a certain line of treatment, does not necessarily denote that it was the result of that particular therapy. Only a successful reproduction of the disease in animal experiments would convince them that the clinical findings claimed, were justified.

Six years had gone since I joined the army, two more than I originally expected to serve. The two additional years following the armistice, which would normally have seen the end of my service, were necessary for me to complete the clinical work on the subject of fluorine. It would have been quite impossible for me to complete it in civilian life. My task accomplished, I was ready to be demobilized, for I had now decided to try experimentally to reproduce in animals the disease which I observed in man. I was hoping that my numerous publications would help me obtain the necessary facilities for further work.

It was already during the war, whilst I was still serving in the army, that I approached the British Medical Research Council to grant me facilities to correlate findings which I obtained in clinical observation in the subject of chronic fluorine poisoning with any findings which might result from animal experiments. I was, however, informed that there would be no chance to make any arrangement with the War Office which would allow me to do such experimental work, but if I cared to apply for assistance after the war, the matter would then receive consideration. The war over, though I was still in uniform, I again asked the Medical Research Council to help me carry out the work. I was advised, however, that it would be necessary for me to take up the question of obtaining facilities for my proposed experimental work with the army authorities, so long as I remained in the Royal Army Medical Corps. After I had been demobilized, it would be open to me to apply to the Medical Research Council for assistance.

On my release from the army, I renewed my request, but in reply I received the following communication: "It is regretted that the Medical Research Council are not in a position to provide you with the accommodation and facilities you require. If, however, you were able to make your own arrangements in this respect, it would be open to you to apply for a research grant in aid of a specific programme of work submitted to the Council for approval."

The highest authorities in the country must have already for some time been cognizant of the hazard to health arising from the ingestion of articles of food and drink contaminated by fluorine. A government-sponsored Inter-Departmental Committee on Food Standards was set up, whose report to the Ministry of Food concluded with the following recommendations:

"Although not within our terms of reference, we desire to bring to the Ministry's notice the need for further research into the effects of long-continued ingestion of small quantities of fluorine in food. We feel that in the areas of India and elsewhere where fluorosis is endemic, ample material is ready to hand for the investigation of this matter which may well have a considerably greater bearing on the public health than has hitherto been generally realized. We suggest that the Ministry should draw the attention of the Medical Research Council, or other organisations able to arrange for the conduct of research work of this kind, to the desirability in the public interest of a thorough investigation of the effects of fluorine ingestion being undertaken at an early date."

Surely no clearer document has ever left the office of any governmental department. Couched in simple, appealing words, it could not, so I thought, fail to move those responsible for the health of the nation into action at an early date. Since in all my publications I had stressed the fact that Great Britain was amongst the countries where chronic fluorine poisoning was endemic, I felt sure that, in accordance with the recommendations of the Inter-Departmental Committee, the Ministry of Food to which they were addressed would welcome the opportunity to have someone at their disposal, who was anxious to continue research work of this kind.

Although, no doubt, the Medical Research Council must have been fully aware of the utter impossibility of an individual medical man's making his own arrangements to do research work of the kind contemplated, I wrote to the Ministry of Food asking for help in obtaining facilities. In reply, I received the following letter from the Scientific Adviser's Division, Ministry of Food:

"I have to tell you that it is not within the province of the Ministry of Food to support medical research of this kind. It is clear from your letter that you have already been in touch with the appropriate authority, and I am afraid that it is not possible for the Ministry of Food to do anything further."

I went from pillar to post in quest of a research institution that would be interested in my work. Amongst them was a Unit of the Medical Research Council doing research work on human nutrition, whose chief appeared to be impressed with what I told him about my program of work, as well as with my publications. He expressed his willingness to allocate for me in his institute the little space necessary to accommodate a few cages of experimental rats. He remarked on parting, however, that as an act of courtesy, he would have to discuss the matter with the secretary of the Medical Research Council, who had jurisdiction over his unit.

Having gained some insight into the methods employed by the Medical Research Council in the control of medical research, I had my qualms over the outcome of that discussion. I was, therefore, not in the least surprised when three weeks later I received the following letter from the chief of the research unit:

"Certain calls on the accommodation in my Unit have been made, which I am under obligation to fulfil, and I am afraid that I cannot arrange the necessary space for you here. I am sorry to have to make this decision and hope that you will be able to find somewhere where you can continue your investigations."

I had not the slightest grudge against the writer of this letter which, I felt, was not written on his own volition. I realized at the same time that its contents fitted exactly into system laid down by those in charge of medical research. The final decision as to which medical subject will be allowed to be investigated rested entirely with one man only, and if he had resolved that the subject was a closed book, however important the subject and whatever the recommendation of an Inter-Departmental Committee, nobody was ever to be permitted to reopen it. In the case of fluorine, this would apparently only apply to an investigation into its effect on the teeth, even if facilities for the latter would have been granted to a distinguished layman with unrestricted connexions with the Council.

When my request for facilities was turned down by a few more institutes, I saw my hopes of ever being able to carry out the proposed experiments dwindle to nothing. As a last resort, however, I approached the Department of Physiology, Middlesex Hospital Medical School, University of London, the hospital at which many years ago I did some post-graduate work, and asked to be granted permission to carry out animal experiments on the systemic effects of long-continued administration of fluorine.

I wish to place on record that of all the men in responsible positions whom I approached for help, only Professor Samson Wright, the head of that Department of Physiology, recognized the importance of the proposed work and placed the necessary space in his animal house at my disposal. I realized that, following the successful completion of my clinical investigation of the problem of fluorine on man, this was the second great chance in my medical career. If successful, the outcome of my experiments could not fail to have an important bearing on further medical developments.

Chapter 15: Experimental Rats Given Fluorine In Their Drinking Water

The animal house at the Department of Physiology, Middlesex Hospital Medical School, is, like that at any other research institute, smaller than an average living room. Stands are fitted against the walls and in the centre of the room, and on top of them are placed cages housing the animals. The cages are marked with the name of the research workers carrying out their experiments.

Mrs. Bee is the undisputed mistress of the animal house, and she keeps her eye on everybody — research workers, staff, and animals. For the past 30 years she has been in charge of her animals, and she speaks of them as one speaks of one's children. She makes sure that everything is kept spotlessly clean and that there is plenty of fresh air in the room. She knows every one of the animals individually, and she would readily recognize and pick out any one amongst the dozen experimental rats housed in the same cage. She is a mother to them all, and she sees to it that they are as happy as possible.

The animals in turn know Mrs. Bee very well. When she returns at feeding time from the market, exhausted from carrying the heavy shopping basket filled with fresh, wholesome food as prescribed for a diet in each particular experiment, they recognized her steps even before they see her enter the room and greet her in unison with a vociferous clamour for food. She commands them to be patient and begins to distribute the rations in the various cages. Quiet is then soon restored.

Rabbits and guinea pigs need no drinking water, their requirements of fluid being fully satisfied by the liquid contained in their food. Since rats, however, must be supplied with drinking water, Mrs. Bee makes sure that the chemical substance ordered to be added to it for experimental purposes is prepared competently in the adjoining preparation room in the exact concentrations required.

Her close collaboration with the research worker is thus indispensable, and she is supported in her responsible position by a staff whose help is as important and reliable as is her own. They are all intimately connected with each experiment and form a team on whose co-operation the outcome of the experiment will ultimately depend.

Outside the staff, nobody has access to the animal house. To maintain the high reputation of the institute, there must not be the slightest interference with the course of the experiment. The handling of the animals is the prerogative of Mrs. Bee and her assistant alone and by the special way in which she fastens the lid of a cage, she is able to tell at a glance whether any unauthorized person has tampered with the animals. This applies, as I soon found out to my great satisfaction, to the research worker himself. When on one occasion in her absence I myself unfastened the lid of one of the cages housing my animals, in order closely to inspect one of them with a magnifying glass for a minute or two, and after replacing it re-fastened the lid of the cage in a manner which must have been different from her own, I was promptly found out and severely reprimanded. This is as it should be. Being now fully conscious of the possibility that the findings obtained might one day be disputed by sceptical critics, I henceforth insisted on having as many witnesses as possible at every step taken in the course of the experiments. Whenever any major developments occurred, the chief of the department, who throughout the experiment supervised it in a general manner, was specially informed. In addition, in the course of the experiments the help of other departments such as X-ray, pathology, biochemistry, photography, etc., had to be invited. The experiments were, therefore, an open book to all those placed in responsible positions at the hospital.

When I first met Mrs. Bee in the office of the head of the department to discuss the plan of action, she gave me a scrutinizing look to find out what kind of man she would have to deal with. In the course of her long reign at the animal house she had met a good many research workers, all of them at the beginning very enthusiastic about the prospects of their work, but most of them gradually admitting failure one after another. No wonder she had become sceptical about any new experiment and remarked that nothing to write home about had ever come of the work. Consequently, she must have had her doubts concerning my proposed work as well. She nevertheless promised me her own and her staff's full collaboration, and she kept her promise to the end.

The question to be solved was: Since the clinical picture observed on man was found to be due to the long-continued ingestion of toxic amounts of fluorine, would it be possible to reproduce the disease in experimental animals?

For experimental purposes, the rat is the most convenient animal, particularly because its structure is very similar to that of man. Owing to its ferocity, the rat has a bad reputation. This may be fully justified in the wild variety, but the albino rat is as a rule no less tame a creature than is the albino mouse, a favourite playmate of children. The response of the wild rat is more dependable in laboratory experiments than is that of the white rat, which for many generations has been reared in unnaturally sheltered conditions. Since the wild rat is, however, more difficult to handle, I chose for my experiments the cross-bred black and white rat.

Groups of twelve male rats, four to five weeks old, were placed in each of six cages, and given the ordinary mixed laboratory diet. One of these groups served as "controls", being supplied with ordinary tap water. The remaining five groups had sodium fluoride added to their drinking water to give initial concentrations of 10, 20, 30, 40, and 50 parts per million (p.p.m.) of added fluorine.

The rats were inspected daily, but no change had occurred in any of them after five weeks, either in their physical appearance or in their general behaviour. They remained lively and vigorous, taking their food and drink well. The fluorine concentration in the drinking water was then increased by 10 p.p.m. each week for the following 21 weeks.

Even after ten weeks no changes occurred, except in the animals drinking water, containing; 100 p.p.m. of fluorine, whose teeth at this time regularly became mottled. The teeth of a few rats receiving 60 p.p.m. of fluorine were, however, almost equally affected. As the ingested fluorine concentration increased, the whole surface of the normally mahogany brown teeth became opaque and resembled ivory in appearance.

Such dental changes occurring in the experimental rats as a result of the action of fluorine were already well-known through the experiments of previous workers. In my experiment, however, I found that the statement that whilst a concentration of 1 p.p.m. of fluorine is needed with man to produce mottling of the teeth, a concentration of some 15 p.p.m. is necessary with rats to obtain the same result, did not apply, since not less than a concentration of between 60 and 100 p.p.m. of fluorine in the drinking water was necessary to change the normal colour of the rats' teeth into milk-white or paper-white mottling. This fact is of fundamental importance, inasmuch as it is not the concentration of fluorine in the drinking water (or in any article of food and drink, for that matter), which produces mottling of the teeth in the rat or man, but the sum, total of fluorine ingested with contaminated food and drink in the course of the day, which must be considered. A small quantity of a high concentration of fluorine will act in precisely the same manner as will a large quantity of a low concentration of the poison. The ingestion of fluorine in however small concentration in the drinking water will, therefore, exert a harmful effect with greater certainty during the hot summer months when more water is drunk to quench the thirst than in the cool season.

Even at the risk of repetition, we must never lose sight of the fact that mottling of the teeth is the first visible sign of chronic fluorine poisoning. Its appearance in our experiment was, therefore, the signal for a careful watch for the inevitable further signs of the disease. Soon the animals were affected by frequent yawning. Later there was intense hiccup which on occasions, especially on the days of the weekly increase of the fluorine concentration in the drinking water, became very severe.

As the fluorine concentration was increased in the drinking water, a few rats were afflicted by sores on the skin of various parts of the body and by the presence of mites, followed by changes in the hair. The hairs bristled and could easily be pulled out. When the concentration of fluorine in the drinking water was further increased to the limit of tolerance there was a visible loss of hair, first in small patches all over the body and on the head, but soon turning into pronounced baldness which was very similar in its distribution to that occurring in man.

Later still, several of the rats developed bulging of the eyes, and in one animal a cataract was noticed in one eye. A stage was reached at which the rats with their highly developed sense of smell, became suspicious of the quality of their drinking water when it contained large quantities of the sodium fluoride dissolved in it. To avoid the smell, they approached the drinking tube supplying them with water from underneath, so as to have its opening farther away from their nostrils than if they approached it, as they normally do, in an erect position. On other occasions they were seen to lick greedily the drop or two of water hanging on the outside of the drinking tube, or eagerly to catch each drop in the air as it fell out through the opening of the tube. It was concluded that, contrary to the general belief, sodium fluoride dissolved in water does have a smell, which is perceived in large concentrations by the highly sensitive rat, but not by man.

It was most interesting to watch the psychological reaction of the rats living their community life in one cage to the supply of a drinking water that contained large quantities of fluorine. One or the other amongst them was seen to assume the role of a warden standing guard at the opening of the tube and keeping the rest from partaking of the poisoned water. On a few occasions he was seen to push any of his mates approaching the drinking tube with a gesture very similar to one which a man would make when asking others to keep away because of danger.

This attitude was obviously caused by the presence of large quantities of fluorine in the drinking water. Another curious example of behaviour was occasionally observed amongst the rats subjected to the action of fluorine, but not amongst the "control" animals ingesting drinking water that was not fluoridated. One or other of them was seen to assume the role of a "strong man" domineering the others, swooping down upon them as if attacking. Intimidated, the rest would form a half-circle silently confronting the brute on their hind legs and raising the front legs in the air. A minute or two later the community resumed their habitual life of eating and sleeping. Psychologists would have a fertile field for a study of what the long-continued ingestion of toxic amounts of fluorine is capable of doing to the mind of those particularly susceptible.

As the experiment proceeded, a stage was reached in the concentration of fluorine in the drinking water at which some of the rats died either from dehydration due to their refusal to drink the poisoned water or from the direct effect of its long-continued ingestion. It was to be expected that the surviving animals would soon die in the same manner.

Chapter 16: Life And Health Of Fluoridated Rats Are Saved By Pure Drinking Water And Calcium

The research worker in his laboratory has to be guided above all by strict objectiveness of observation. In no circumstances must he allow himself to be carried away by enthusiasm and to become biased one way or the other. The observations he makes must be based on facts, not on fancy.

So far, the animal experiment had definitely shown that apart from mottling of the teeth the rats developed a severe skin disease which was accompanied by loss of hair, and that as the concentration of fluorine added to the drinking water was increased they drank as little of it as was necessary to satisfy their indispensable requirements of fluids. Some of the animals died, either because of the effect of fluorine already ingested or because they refused to drink the water altogether and became dehydrated.

So as to save the remaining rats for further work the experiment had to be interrupted, and the fluoridated water was replaced by plain tap water. The response of the rats was striking — the animals at once rushed to the new water supply. A fierce struggle developed, and finally as many as four animals in a cage managed to settle down to drink simultaneously from one tube. A short interval of not more than 10 days was sufficient to restore their vitality in a remarkable degree. The hair became smooth again, the skin turned normal and there was a complete regrowth of hair over the denuded areas.

Resumption of the original experiment, however, caused recurrence of the condition. A few of the rats developed severe eczema on various parts of the body, accompanied by renewed loss of hair. Moreover, the ear lobes underwent grave changes: They lost their normal outline, they became thickened and ragged, and they looked as if torn into shreds, each of which was studded with numerous excrescences in a cauliflower fashion. Mites were observed on and around the sores on the skin. Because of its similarity to rat leprosy, the condition is in our textbooks referred to as "the leprosy-like disease of the rat", and attributed to a highly contagious infestation by mites. The rats so affected are said to be of no further use for experimentation.

This would mean that the lesions of the skin and hair observed had nothing to do with the experiment. It would signify the end of a work so far extended over a period of many months. The animals would have to be sacrificed.

At this juncture, however, I remembered that the experimental removal, already described on a previous occasion, of the parathyroid glands·in rats some 45 years ago in Vienna, ended in precisely the same manner. It was at that time stated that mites had invaded the skin of the animals and had produced severe sores from which they died.

Surely, I told Mrs. Bee, before sacrificing the poor animals it would be worth our while to see whether, in spite of what the textbooks say, these grave lesions on the skin, hair and ear lobes have really nothing to do with fluorine. Let us see, I said, what happens to the rats if we give them treatment directed against the action of that poison. Let us replace the fluoridated drinking water by distilled water and add large quantities of calcium to their food so as to replace that amount of calcium which, we know, fluorine would have removed from their bodies. If we fail — well, we will have to admit defeat, pack up and terminate the experiment.

Mrs. Bee, sceptical as ever, looked incredulous but stuck to her promise to co-operate. Our surprise was great when we saw that within 24 hours of this treatment the warts and nodules on the ear lobes fell off, leaving a sore base underneath. After four weeks, the ear lobes became normal, the nasty sores on various parts of the body were healed completely, and the hair grew again on a normal skin. There were no more mites to be seen.

Obviously, there could be no doubt that, contrary to what was written in the textbooks on diseases affecting the rat, the grave skin lesions were due to nothing but the action of fluorine and that the invasion by mites on a skin which was deprived of calcium was secondary in character.

Yet, always conscious of the probability that even now some incorrigibly disbelieving critics would have some misgivings concerning the correctness of these findings, I had to guard against the possibility of any error. Having succeeded once in first producing and then repairing damage inflicted on experimental rats by giving them fluoridated water to drink for some time and then replacing it by sound water, might it not be possible to do it a second time on the same animals?

One rat, which was cured from the so-called "leprosy-like disease", was once more submitted to the action of fluoridated drinking water. Promptly the nodules and wart-like excrescences re-appeared on the earlobes, but vanished as promptly when treatment directed against fluorine was instituted. In another rat improvement proceeded satisfactorily until it was noticed that for some reason food to which calcium has been added was rejected. The condition on the ear lobes fluctuated, dependent on whether or not calcium was ingested on some days. It was at this point suggested that the lesions described were only indirectly due to the action of fluorine, inasmuch as fluorine had damaged the mucous membrane of the rats' stomach and intestine to such an extent that food could not be properly absorbed.

It was further suggested that the diet on which the animals were fed may have been initially poor in vitamin content. The condition might thus be attributed to vitamin deficiency rather than to the action of fluorine.

Vitamin deficiency is known to cause certain skin lesions, and it has also been observed that children who are fed on a diet poor in vitamins are more liable to have their teeth mottled by the long-continued ingestion of fluorine than are well-fed children.

To find out how vitamins would influence the action of fluorine, a new experiment was carried out. It consisted of the addition of vitamin B to the food of rats which were given fluoridated water to drink. This resulted in the prevention of skin lesions and of loss of hair, which occurred in the previous experiment, when no vitamin B was added to the food. It was concluded that, since the addition of vitamin B to the food of rats, which were given fluoridated water to drink, had a favourable influence on the course of chronic fluorine poisoning, fluorine interferes with the mechanism through which vitamin B exerts its influence on the body.

In the course of these experiments, which took four years to complete, certain organs of the experimental animals were examined under the microscope. It was to be expected that fluorine, like any other potent poison, would severely damage various organs within the body, some of them more than others, but it was necessary to find out to what extent the damage occurred and to demonstrate it to those in the medical profession who are competent to assess it from the pathological point of view.

Several investigators had reported in the past that the organs most damaged by the action of fluorine were the stomach and the intestine, particularly that part which is the continuation of the stomach and is called the duodenum. According to them, the mucous membrane of the digestive canal is red, inflamed and swollen in chronic fluorine poisoning, and gastric and duodenal ulcers develop, some of which penetrate the mucous membrane. These lesions are closely similar to those seen in chronic arsenical poisoning. In my experiments these lesions were absent, probably owing to the fact that the action of fluorine was induced very slowly.

The next organs most frequently affected in chronic fluorine poisoning are the kidneys. In my experiments, the kidneys underwent very severe changes, in every respect identical with those seen in man as a result of Bright's disease.

The thyroid gland, too, was damaged to such an extent that it was difficult to identify the organ under the microscope as the thyroid gland.

The testicles degenerated to such a degree that they could be regarded as having to all intents and purposes disappeared altogether.

The thyroid gland and the testicles belong, together with the parathyroid glands and the adrenals, which on a previous occasion had already been shown clinically to be affected by the action of fluorine, to that vitally important group of glands called the endocrine system. Without their proper functioning health does not exist; when they are severely damaged, death is inevitable.

The endocrine glands, as well as all the organs within the body, including the stomach and intestine, the kidneys, the heart, etc., are supplied by the vegetative nervous system. The vegetative nervous system is entirely independent of our will and acts on its own. It has its origin at the base of the brain, and in its course divides into separate bundles of nerve supply, to be distributed in the various organs.

Not all the bundles are affected by fluorine simultaneously, however. Since the vitality of any one organ depends on, among other factors, the normal condition of the nerve supply, it becomes obvious that the organ is bound to be severely affected if its nerve supply is affected by fluorine. In the case of the stomach and the duodenum, the mucous membrane becomes devitalized and an ulcer develops. In the case of the kidneys, in addition to the involvement of their nerve supply, the greatest part of the fluorine ingested passes through them before being eliminated and irritates them to such an extent over a number of years as to cause Bright's disease. In the case of the heart, the frequent co-existence of low blood pressure with other signs and symptoms of chronic fluorine poisoning has already been mentioned as indicating that the heart muscle becomes soft and flabby and degenerated. Further investigation is sure to throw more light on the question as to what further damage fluorine is capable of producing in other organs of the body.

Chapter 17 Gastric And Duodenal Ulcers And Bright's Disease Caused By Fluorine

When I left London to join the British army, I had not considered that by so doing I might sacrifice an important part of my established medical career. On my release I had to try to recover the lost ground and to pick up at least some of the threads broken by the events of the war. I had no regrets, however, since the study of the problem of fluorine had to take precedence over everything else.

I was soon called to see a man who stated that for the past two years he had suffered from frequent attacks of abdominal colicky pain, which were not relieved by any of the numerous medicines hitherto prescribed. Examination suggested the possibility that the trouble might be due to a duodenal ulcer. X-ray examination revealed the presence not only of a small duodenal, but also of a large gastric ulcer, which radiologically presented the appearance of suspected malignant degeneration. In agreement with the radiologist, dietetic treatment was instituted, and it was decided that, for purposes of comparison, X-ray examination should be repeated in a few weeks time.

Since it is a definitely established fact that long-continued ingestion of fluorine is capable of producing gastric and duodenal ulcers, and also in view of the possibility that in this patient the gastric ulcer might already have undergone a malignant change, the regime usually adopted in cases of ulcer was combined with treatment directed against chronic fluorine poisoning, particularly since the combined treatment could in no circumstances harm the patient.

The second X-ray examination, which was carried out by the same radiologist after five weeks' treatment, revealed that both the gastric and the duodenal ulcers had healed completely, without leaving a trace. This finding fully harmonized with the greatly improved condition of the patient.

In the course of my medical career I have seen a large number of patients suffering from gastric and duodenal ulceration, but in none of them was the success of treatment carried out on orthodox lines as promptly and as completely as it was in the present case, when the possibility of fluorine was taken into account as a contributory, if not the sole, cause of the illness.

It has already been pointed out that, next to the gastrointestinal tract, the kidneys are the organ most frequently affected by fluorine. Even before I joined the British Army, an opportunity was afforded me to investigate whether findings concerning damage to the kidneys, which occurs with great regularity in experimental fluorine poisoning in animals, as well as in fatal cases of acute fluorine intoxication following suicidal, homicidal or accidental ingestion of large doses of fluorine in man, could be utilized in the treatment of a severe case of Bright's disease.

A young man, whom for several years I had known as the healthy and robust son accompanying his ailing mother when she came to see me in my consulting room, became the unfortunate victim of Bright's disease. He was admitted first to one, then to another hospital, both of which he left improved, but each time the condition recurred soon after. When I saw him, he was extremely ill and a cure by any method of treatment seemed beyond the realm of possibility. His broken-hearted mother, however, hoped that a miracle could be accomplished by a renewed attempt at saving her son. More from a desire to console her and to soothe her sorrow, even if only for the brief remainder of her son's pitiable life, than in hope that it might be successful, I prescribed treatment, directed against chronic fluorine poisoning.

Ordinarily I would have expected the mother to ring me up in the course of the following few days to tell me how things were going on, and when I heard nothing I assumed that everything was over. I still remember, however, my great surprise when about a fortnight later she rang me up to inform me how very much better her son was, and to ask me to see him again. When I saw him, I could not trust my own eyes. The man was still ill but he was very considerably better than he had been only a fortnight ago and was defying the prognostication of all the medical men, including myself, who had seen him in the course of his long-drawn out illness. Immediately the old saying entered my mind: "While there is life, there is hope." I asked him to carry on with the treatment and to continue his strict rest in bed. Laughing, he replied that he never went to bed, but that "he took it easy". Not more than another fortnight later, altogether four weeks after the treatment had begun, the man was to all intents and purposes restored to active life.

On my demobilization, the mother informed me that her son had remained quite well for about 6 years following this treatment. He was even well enough to volunteer for service during the war on the home front with the Ambulance Corps. After the war, however, he had a recurrence of his illness to which he succumbed.

Not only do these two cases of gastric and duodenal ulceration on the one hand of Bright's disease on the other tally perfectly with what is generally accepted as being capable of being reproduced in experimental animals by the administration of fluorides, but the result of treatment aiming at their removal from the body must be looked upon as yet another successful outcome of the "therapeutic test". It indicates that fluorine was the cause, or at any rate a contributing factor, in producing these two common diseases in mankind.

It will, however, again be objected by sceptical critics that no such definite, far-reaching conclusions are justifiable so long as only one case each of these serious illnesses has been submitted to treatment directed against the action of fluorine. They would insist on having confirmatory reports from various sources on numerous cases of the kind. This is indeed a very legitimate criticism, one which will, however, be tempered by the fact that whatever the number of cases required as a basis for final judgment, that number must necessarily start with unit one. It is up to those responsible for advancing medical knowledge in the interest of mankind to see to it that numerous cases of recurrent gastric and duodenal ulceration, of Bright's disease, and of cancer in any part of the body, be submitted to the "therapeutic test" directed against the action of fluorine.

In the vast majority of cases, treatment of gastric and duodenal ulcers is medical and is carried out for a long time before the question of surgical intervention arises. In far advanced cases of Bright's disease, the patient is invariably admitted to a hospital for treatment. As far as cancer in any part of the body is concerned, in the state of our present knowledge, operation becomes imperative at the earliest possible moment after the diagnosis is made. Unfortunately, however, there are all over the world numerous cases of cancer which were not operated on in time and which consequently became inoperable. Many millions of money are expended every year in support of institutions in which the poor victims of chronic incurable diseases have to spend the few remaining years of their miserable existence. These are the patients on whom the "therapeutic test" extended over a sufficient length of time should be carried out, because of the possibility that their condition may have been caused by the action of fluorine. The treatment is simple and involves only a few dietary changes and the administration of certain medicines. To stand any chance of success, however, this treatment should be carried out under the supervision of the medical and nursing staff of the institution, so as to make sure that all the sources of further intake of fluorine are cut off, and that the few medicines aimed at counteracting the effect of the amounts of the poison accumulated in the body over a number of years are administered in accordance with the instructions. Apart from a few restrictions, there would be no need whatsoever for the inmates of those institutions to alter the mode of life hitherto adopted. In fact, the chief changes would fall on the shoulders of the kitchen personnel.

To turn these ideas into action, I approached Professor R. W. Scarff, Director of the Bland-Sutton Institute of Pathology, Middlesex Hospital, London, in his capacity as Secretary of the British Empire Cancer Campaign, with a view to obtaining his help in promoting the project. Professor Scarff agreed that, although an enormous amount of laboratory work was going on all over the world, nothing has so far been done to bridge the wide gap in our knowledge of the true nature of cancer by means of the proposed clinical investigation. He promised to help me, if I succeeded in finding a hospital for cases of cancer, for which medically nothing further can be done, that would grant facilities for the contemplated treatment. He sent me to the Lady Almoner of the Middlesex Hospital who gave me a list of the institutions to which such cases were referred by the hospital.

I communicated with but was refused by all of these institutions on the grounds either that their facilities were so limited and cramped that they could not possibly engage in any additional undertaking, or that it would be quite impracticable to alter the patients' standard diet in the way that would be necessary to carry out the treatment, because the cook would give notice and leave on account of the additional work.

There was around that time a lively discussion in Great Britain about the case of an osteopath who claimed to have discovered an unfailing method of curing cancer. It was only under great pressure that the discoverer agreed to demonstrate his method of treatment to medical experts. When his request for an opportunity to prove his case was rejected, he invited the help of a member of Parliament to raise the matter in the House of Commons. The House of Commons convened a committee of the highest medical authorities to investigate the matter, and the Minister of Health, Mr. Aneurin Bevan, wrote an encouraging letter to the osteopath.

Emboldened by the contents of that letter, which was publicized in the daily press, I assumed that, although a member of the medical profession with which Mr. Bevan was perpetually at loggerheads over the question of Socialized Medicine, I was entitled to hope that my own work on the subject of chronic fluorine poisoning and its possible connexion which the cancer problem would be investigated by a committee of medical authorities of not lesser standing than were those in the case of the osteopath. I wrote Mr. Bevan a letter in which I asked for facilities to carry out treatment directed against the action of fluorine on victims of inoperable cancer and enclosed reprints of my medical publications. The following was the reply from the Ministry of Health:

"I am directed by the Minister of Health to say that your letter of the 12th October, 1950, and its enclosures, have been studied with interest, but that the Minister is not in a position to select individual new projects for research, nor can he make available patients for trial of unproven methods of treatment. He suggests that your best course would be to approach individual centres where research is carried out with a view to obtaining further investigation of your ideas, which do not appear yet to have received practical trial."

The approach of individual centres where research is carried out elicited, as we now know, the information that the proposed investigation could not be permitted because of the risk that cook would give notice and leave, owing to additional duties in the kitchen.

Chapter 18: Actions Of Fluorine And Arsenic Identical.

As we now know, the gradual development of our knowledge of what fluorine is capable of doing to mankind started with the realization that various complaints made by a large number of people about indifferent health suggested some kind of poisoning caused by an unknown substance. As the study of the disease advanced, the impression gained ground that the poisoning was very similar to that produced by the slow action of arsenic. This impression was based mainly on the presence of digestive trouble, on attacks of neuralgiae which were more frequent in the legs than in the arms, and on the co-existence of skin eruptions. Was this then, it was asked, a repetition of the notorious epidemic of arsenical poisoning which occurred at the beginning of the present century in the Midlands, England, and assumed such proportions that a Royal Commission was appointed to make a thorough inquiry into its causes and recommend methods of its prevention in the future? As a result of that inquiry, legislation was set up to prohibit the use of arsenical preparations in food and drink, thereby making another outbreak of an epidemic of arsenical poisoning most unlikely.

The methods of detecting even slight traces of arsenic in the various materials collected from the victim of the disease are reliable. Since in the present occurrence of chronic illness no traces of arsenic could be found to account for it, it was concluded that another substance might be at work, which in its action was very similar to that of arsenic. The close similarity between the action of arsenic and that of the other substance, which subsequently proved to be fluorine, is manifest from the attached table. The list of signs and symptoms encountered in chronic arsenical poisoning was taken from current medical textbooks and is familiar to every student of Medicine.

SYMPTOM	ARSENIC	FLORINE
Constipation	Alternating With Diarrhoea	Present
Severe gas formation	Not Quoted	Present
Neuritis and Neuralgiae	Present	Present
Tender Calves	Present	Present
Irritation of the skin, "pins and needles", deadness and numbness in hands and fingers	Present	Present
Frequent attacks of "common cold", running nose, sneezing, sore throat	Present	Present
Hoarseness, huskiness of voice	Present	Present
Bronchitis, catarrh of upper air passages	Present	Present
Conjunctivitis, lachrymation	Present	Present
Bleeding of the gums	Present	Present
Excessive salivation, dribbling at the corner of the mouth	Present	Present
Disturbances of hearing	Present	Present
Excessive perspiration	Present	Present
Skin eruptions, eczema	Present	Present
Hardening of the skin on the palms and soles	Present	Present
Warts	Present	Present
Mottling of the teeth	Not Quoted	Present
Loss of hair	Present	Present
Changes in the finger- and toe-nails	Present	Present
White specks and lines on the nails	Not Quoted	Present
Brown patches on the skin	Present	Present
General weakness and tiredness	Present	Present
Varicose veins	Not Quoted	Present
Swelling of the legs	Present	Present
Mental disturbances	Present	Present

These being the facts of the situation, I was bold enough to assume that no medical man worth his salt could possibly, on becoming cognizant of them, be content with sitting back and waiting for others to take the initiative for further work on the subject. Such an attitude of "laissez faire" would inevitably lead mankind to lose confidence in a profession which was in duty bound to have matters rectified without any further loss of time.

A stage had now been reached in which all the preparatory work carried out over a number of years appeared to have been completed, so that the findings obtained could be put to practical application for the benefit of humanity. Having failed, at any rate for the time being, to obtain facilities at a hospital for inoperable cases of cancer because of alleged difficulties in the kitchen arrangements, I decided to turn elsewhere.

The frequent occurrence in the course of chronic fluorine poisoning of lesions in organs originating in the ectoderm, namely the skin and its appendages, the teeth, nails and hair, is now an established fact. It has been shown that they are brought about through fluorine attacking, via the general blood circulation, the peripheral and the vegetative nervous systems which supply the various organs of the body. It has also been emphasized that fluorine has a predilection for the nervous tissue. By affecting the nervous system primarily, it produces secondary damage in the organs supplied. Moreover, like the skin and its appendages, the nervous system also has its origin in the ectoderm during intra-uterine life.

Pursuing the problem of fluorine in all its implications, it was impossible to leave out of account the obvious fact that the brain itself is part of the nervous system. Together with the spinal cord, it constitutes the central nervous system, on whose proper functioning life itself depends. How, I asked myself, could the brain, or any other organ of the body for that matter, escape damage whilst it was nourished by blood that contained toxic amounts of fluorine? The frequent fits of depression and melancholia alternating with irritability, the forgetting of recent events, the difficulty in finding the right word to express a thought, the gloomy outlook on life without adequate reason; all suggested that the mind of the victims of chronic fluorine poisoning is affected to some extent.

The favourable result of treatment directed against the effects of the poison, which was obtained both in man and in experimental animals, emboldened me to assume that it would be worthwhile to investigate whether fully developed mental diseases could not be influenced in a like manner. I approached the superintendent of a large mental hospital on the outskirts of London for help in the matter. He invited me to address the entire staff of the hospital in

91

order to acquaint them with my past work and to outline my plans for the proposed investigation. Amongst the results of my work achieved, I spoke of the disturbance of pigmentation occurring in the course of chronic fluorine poisoning, and I showed slides depicting the case of "the brown girl", as it appeared before and after treatment. My aim, I explained, was to see whether certain forms of mental disease would not give way to identical treatment, which I would be happy to carry out under the fullest supervision of the hospital staff

In the discussion that followed a member of the staff stated that in his experience there was a frequent co-existence of disturbed pigmentation in mental diseases. There were in his ward two women who had a pigmentation on the face and other parts of the body, which was very similar to the one of "the brown girl". This was of particular interest to me because, although till then I knew nothing of such co-existence, it confirmed what I had assumed as a possibility on theoretical grounds. I suggested that it would be advisable first of all to make a survey of inmates of the hospital, suffering from whatever form of mental illness, without my knowing beforehand the diagnosis, who, in addition to patches of brown skin, exhibited some of the ectodermal lesions as external visible signs of chronic fluorine poisoning.

A short time later I received the following letter from this physician:

"With reference to your recent visit to this hospital when you discussed the possibilities of fluorine being an aetiological agent in mental diseases, I mentioned to you that I thought we had such a case in this hospital. I have since started her on treatment and she appears to be improving. I also examined a number of chronic patients for fluorine stigmata. A very large percentage have one or more of the stigmata you quote in your articles.

I would be extremely grateful if you could find time to give me clearer guidance as to what is considered to be adequate evidence of poisoning. It is pointed out that no aluminium utensils are used in cooking in the hospital kitchens. Will this factor prevent the maintenance of toxic levels of fluorine being sustained in patients who have been in the hospital for considerable periods?

I would add that I was very interested in your discussion and would be only too glad to cooperate in any investigations you wish to carry out."

The letter coming, as it did, from a younger member of the medical profession is quoted verbatim in support of the contention that there still exists a spirit of healthy idealism in Medicine. I emphatically reject the view that this spirit is to be found only amongst the young members of the profession whilst engaged in hospital work. I gave the writer of the letter all the information required, and told him in particular that not using aluminium utensils in the kitchen of the hospital would not in the slightest influence my views on the subject, since the mental illness originated before the patient was admitted to the hospital, when most likely she did use aluminium cooking utensils at home over a number of years; because aluminium kitchen utensils, though an important source of supply of toxic amounts of fluorine in food, were by no means the only one in view of the fact that everyday articles of food and drink themselves contained fluorine to add to those which were accumulated in the body for a long time; and also because it was essential for the success of the treatment not only to cut off, as far as possible, every further intake of fluorine, but also to eliminate from the body those quantities which, whilst there, continued to exert their harmful effect.

I have seen the patient referred to in the letter and found on her a facial pigmentation as pronounced as was that of "the brown girl". I have watched her progress at weekly intervals. After not more than three months of treatment, the facial pigmentation disappeared altogether, and the mental condition became normal, so that she was discharged from the hospital as cured.

I should add that although it was very difficult to apply treatment on this patient in the ward, in which she was living with other patients who were not subjected to the dietary precautions, I was informed that she had collaborated with the nursing staff to the full. I will further add that, whilst the outstandingly, favourable outcome of the treatment on this patient, who spent some three years at the hospital, was being discussed, it was suddenly remembered that a year ago she was submitted to lobotomy, a brain operation carried out in the treatment of mental illness which sometimes shows a beneficial result only after the lapse of as many as 12 months. The present undoubted cure, it was argued, might therefore be attributable to the operation rather than to the treatment directed against chronic fluorine poisoning. No explanation could, however, be obtained for the simultaneous disappearance of the facial pigmentation.

There was yet another patient in the same ward, whose face and other parts of the body were likewise pigmented. The same treatment was applied, but although both the mental condition and the pigmentation showed signs of improvement, no cure was obtainable owing to lack of co-operation on the part of the patient.

Chapter 19: Case Of Nerve-Leprosy Is Associated With Chronic Fluorine Poisoning

My suggestion for a survey amongst the inmates of the hospital who exhibited both disturbance of pigmentation of the skin and ectodermal lesions was accepted. Before starting the examination, I requested that the nature of the mental illness should not be disclosed to me until afterwards. Some 25 male patients, about one-half of those inspected, were selected for treatment. The external manifestations of chronic fluorine poisoning varied in degree and extent. I was, however, deeply impressed by the subsequent information that most of those amongst the patients selected, who had patches of brown skin and ectodermal lesions simultaneously in a marked degree, were suffering from schizophrenia.

It was, in my view, essential that the patients selected should be segregated in a separate ward, so as to make it easier for a special nurse allotted to see to it that the treatment was carried out in a proper manner under the supervision of the physician-in-charge. Without this precaution, the program would be doomed to failure. The shortage of nursing staff prevailing since the end of the war in this as in other hospitals was known to me, and the superintendent, who at all times expressed his desire to be helpful, described the position accurately when he wrote me the following letter:

"Dr. C. confirms your opinion that in regard to his two cases the physical signs which you attribute to Riehl's Melanosis" (brown pigmentation of the face and the neck) "certainly cleared up on the regime which you prescribed, but for various reasons of which you are aware, it is impossible to draw any conclusions in regard to the mental state of these cases. C. tells me he has another similar case now."

"I had a chat with Dr. H about your carrying out the treatment on some of his cases, but H. says it is frankly impossible to do this work in the male wards at the present time owing to the extreme shortage of male nurses. It requires a great deal of nursing supervision to ensure that the treatment is being properly carried out, and it seems physically impossible for us to obtain this at the present time. Thus, as I see it, although willing to offer you every facility, my medical colleagues here seem to be limited to apply the treatment to not more than one or two cases at a time."

The phrase "various reasons of which you are aware" that made it impossible to draw any conclusions in regard to the mental state, referred to the operation of lobotomy, which had been performed on one of the two patients a year before the facial pigmentation and the mental illness cleared up simultaneously in the course of treatment directed against chronic fluorine poisoning. As it was, I reluctantly came to the conclusion that nothing would be gained, even if I were to succeed in one or two more cases under the unfavourable conditions described. I realized that so far as obtaining practical results was concerned, I had failed once more — at any rate for the time being.

I say "for the time being" designedly. Since my release from the army I had achieved no practical results which would directly, and as I thought, immediately benefit suffering humanity. It became obvious to me that, as time went on, my chances of continuing my work would decrease rather than improve in an environment in which, following the havoc of war, research was at a low ebb. I therefore decided to take a step even more drastic than the one I took when I left London some years previously to join the army in order to investigate the problem of mottling of the teeth due to the action of fluorine. Being unable to pursue my work in England, I would try to find facilities elsewhere.

I knew that my publications were known and appreciated in the United States but were ignored in Great Britain. The problem of fluorine had its cradle in the United States, and interest in medical progress had not suffered through the events of the war. On the contrary, what Europe had lost during the past 20 years, the United States had gained in increasing medical knowledge. I therefore decided to transfer my search for a practical solution of the problem of certain chronic diseases which I believed might be due to the long-continued ingestion of toxic amounts of fluorine to the United States. True, I did not know anybody there who would be able to help me, but I felt there was enough "life in the old dog yet" for a new adventure in the New World.

Before leaving the Old Country, in which I had spent 30 years of my life, I would have dearly loved to investigate one more condition, which might have some connexion with the subject of fluorine. In my experiments described in a previous chapter, some of the rats which were given gradually increasing doses of sodium fluoride in their drinking water developed lesions attributed to "the leprosy-like disease of the rat". I succeeded in proving that, contrary to the general belief, the disease was not contagious or due to infestation by mites, but was caused by the long-continued action of fluorine. On withholding fluorine and on the addition of calcium to the food, the disease was eradicated.

The lesions on the ear lobes of the animals suffering from "the leprosy-like disease of the rats" were closely similar to those encountered in human leprosy. Was there any possibility fluorine, which is a nerve-poison pure and simple, was the cause of that variety of human leprosy known as "nerve leprosy"? An extensive study of human leprosy revealed the fact that several signs and symptoms are common to both this disease and chronic fluorine poisoning. In both certain nerves, particularly the ulnar nerve already mentioned on a previous page, are affected, producing the sensation of "pins and needles" and deadness and numbness in the fingers and hands. Loss of hair, changes in the finger- and toe-nails, disturbance of pigmentation, and an abnormal reaction of the vegetative nervous system, occur in both of them. Both human leprosy and chronic fluorine poisoning are favourably influenced by large doses of calcium. Further study of human leprosy revealed the fact that already some 50 years ago a great British physician, Sir Jonathan Hutchinson, after a carefully conducted investigation extended over various parts of the British dominions formed the opinion that leprosy might be caused by a poison ingested with some kind of food. He thought that the poison might be something quite different from Hansen's bacillus, which is believed to be the cause of leprosy, and that it might be of a chemical nature.

During the intervening months of waiting for the permit of entry into the United States I was anxious to investigate in a practical manner whether treatment directed against chronic fluorine poisoning would in any way influence the course of leprosy, particularly in children. This would constitute another "therapeutic test", and would throw considerable light on the problem, if carried out in a leprosarium housing large numbers of the unfortunate victims of the disease.

With the invaluable help of the British Foreign Office, I succeeded in communicating with the chief of the National Leprosarium in Tokyo, Japan, with a view to obtaining facilities for my proposed work. I sent him reprints of my publications on the subject of chronic fluorine poisoning, which would form the basis for my proposed project, and received the following reply:

"From studying your thesis, I believe that your research on fluorine poisoning will throw a new light on the treatment of leprosy. Therefore, I am most willing to be of any assistance to you if after coming here and seeing our patients you care to utilize your studies in this treatment. We welcome you most heartily, and I am eagerly looking forward to rendering my services for your work."

Owing to the exigencies of the post-war period, however, my request for entry clearance into Japan, addressed to the highest military authorities, came to nothing.

Still undaunted by the failure to attain my object, I began to look out for cases of leprosy in London. Soon one was found at a hospital, in which the diagnosis of "nerve-leprosy" was fully established. The physician-in-charge, who knew of my interest in the disease, turned the patient over to me and left us together. He was, however, not more than four or five paces away when I had to recall him and to invite him to have a look at the patient's teeth. A simple glance at them revealed at once that they were all markedly mottled, thus showing that during the first 8 years of the patient's life he had ingested toxic amounts of fluorine. Further investigation elicited the fact that the first sign of what later proved to be "nerve-leprosy" were noticed by the patient at the age of 9 years, and might well have been present earlier. Several additional examinations disclosed further evidence of the action of fluorine. Its presence in his nails and hair, which has been detected by chemical analysis, indicated that the poison was accumulated in his body.

As far as I know, this is the first record of a case of "nerve-leprosy" associated with chronic fluorine poisoning. One swallow does not make a summer, however, and it must be left to further research to find out whether the two conditions are identical.

Chapter 20: I Plan Further Research

As zero hour came into sight, I desired, in order to save time, to make long-range preparations for my proposed work in the United States. Any attempt to make my own arrangements for further investigation on arrival in the country would, to judge by my past experience, prove futile and involve considerable loss of time. The work would have to be sponsored by one of the numerous organizations in existence, whose zeal for medical progress was well-known all over the world, and who would, I thought, do everything in their power to promote a project that promised to be successful. Obviously, they would be guided by recommendations coming from a research institute, a hospital, or an industrial concern having a direct interest in the subject to be explored. In my own case, there was for a stranger no alternative but to approach one of those organizations in a direct manner. In the forefront of these organizations stands the Rockefeller Institute for Medical Research. Its aim is "to conduct, assist and encourage investigations in the sciences and arts of hygiene, medicine and surgery, and allied subjects, in the nature and causes of disease and the methods of its prevention and treatment, and to make knowledge relating to these various subjects available for the protection of the health of the public and the improved treatment of disease and injury". These are indeed lofty ideals, worthy of a great civilized country, and their fulfillment is bound in due course to make for a happier life, and for alleviation of suffering and misery of mankind.

Already in 1947, and on my release from the army and before I succeeded in finding facilities for carrying out my animal experiments at the Department of Physiology, Middlesex Hospital Medical School, London, I entertained the idea of going to the United States for the purpose of continuing my work on fluorine, I wrote to the Rockefeller Foundation concerning my plans and enclosed reprints of my publications. The following was the reply:

"I am afraid I do not have any suggestions which are likely to be helpful to you in realizing your wish to carry on your researches in the United States. It is true that there are one or two groups in this country who are pursuing work on the subject of fluorine poisoning but, so far, the Foundation has not gone seriously into the question."

"As a matter of long term policy, the Foundation has always tried to avoid encouraging scientists from other countries to settle permanently here; indeed its interests have always been in the other direction. At the present time it seems more than ever necessary to avoid doing anything which might serve to increase the present grave shortage in Europe of trained medical investigators. We very much hope, therefore, that you can find some way of carrying on your work either in England or better still on the European continent itself. Admittedly the situation there is not encouraging at present but we all hope that something like normal conditions will be restored within the next three or four years."

Though disappointed, I was not dismayed. It would require much more than that to damp my enthusiasm for continued work, and even then it would be only for a short spell of time. Nor was, as far as I knew, the information correct that there were one or two groups who were pursuing work on the subject of fluorine poisoning, unless the writer had biochemical investigation in mind, which was carried out on experimental animals. To my knowledge, there was no study anywhere in the world of the effect of long-continued ingestion of toxic amounts of fluorine in man, as it affects him in everyday life. Having in the meantime found facilities for carrying out my animal experiments, I did not bother to write a letter of thanks for the unsolicited advice given.

Now, four years later, that my plans for emigration were near realization, I wrote the Rockefeller Foundation again asking for facilities for further work, and pointed out that there would be no legal obstacle on that score, since it was my intention to apply for the first citizenship papers and to try to obtain a license to practise Medicine at any hospital in the State of New York. The following was the reply:

"This is to acknowledge the receipt of your letter of June 9, 1951, with your appended curriculum vitae and bibliography of your researches on chronic fluorine poisoning."

"I am very sorry indeed to have to inform you that it is not possible for you to obtain facilities for the further pursuit of your work under the auspices of the Rockefeller Foundation. I might add that I note from your letter that you plan, on your arrival in the United States next October, to take out your first citizenship papers and to attempt to become licensed to practise in New York State. It is certainly a courageous undertaking for a man of your age, 63, to attempt this."

I still was not dismayed, but I will admit that the letter gave me plenty of food for thought. Did then this letter, written by a responsible official in high position, mean to indicate that in the United States a man aged 63 has no right anymore to aspire to "a courageous undertaking" of the type contemplated? If so, it seemed to me that more, not less, medical research was badly needed in the United States to find out the cause of the apparent inferior status forced on men of this age. Worse still, as a result of this and the previous letter emanating from the Rockefeller Institute for Medical Research, I had my doubts as to whether those lofty ideals professed in its aims were to be taken quite literally after all. Yet, all these considerations would not in the slightest deter me from pursuing my plans, come what might.

The time of my departure arrived. The immigration officer on the liner, having found my documents in order, wished me God speed and good luck in the New World. In thanking him, I remarked that I should be in great need of it.

The Statue of Liberty carrying the torch of light and knowledge into every corner of the world came into view as the famed symbol of a land where freedom of thought and expression, and where progress in every field of human endeavour reign supreme, unfettered by red tape and oppressive restrictions. So this was the United States of America where, in spite of certain minor disappointments already encountered, everybody would do his best in support of my work! Gone were the days when, during the war, I required an expert histological examination in an important case connected with my work and, in return, I was requested to share the authorship of a paper, on which I alone spent many months of hard work. When I rejected the preposterous request, I had to use my wits to discover that a specimen taken from a normal person had been substituted for the pathological one which I had submitted for examination, so as to upset the very foundation of my laborious work on the case! Gone were the days when I had to beg a little man in the Department of Biochemistry of a hospital to have a few tests carried out for me, which I thought were vitally important in the investigation of another case. The little man would, of course, be backed up by his equally little superiors, and the tests would have to be omitted. Nor would there be any more necessity for me to deal with those numerous small and still smaller dictators met at every corner of medical research.

I had been only a few days in New York, when I found that great interest was taken in the subject of fluorine throughout the country. When speaking to the man in the street, I realized that he knew a great deal about the problem. For some time reports had reached London from the United States to the effect that, since mottled teeth due to the long-continued ingestion of small quantities of fluorine appeared to be less liable to decay than were teeth which were not mottled, the United States Public Health authorities recommended that fluorides be added to the public water supplies. I first thought this to be a hoax perpetrated on medical science. As time went on, however, it became obvious that it was in all

101

seriousness proposed by those in authority to add as much fluorine to any public water supply as was necessary to make up a concentration of 1.2 p.p.m.

It was with good reason that I had reiterated the statement that it was the ingestion of a drinking water with a concentration as low as 1 p.p.m. of fluorine, which was sufficient to produce mottling of the teeth as the first visible sign of chronic fluorine poisoning. On this statement rests our knowledge of the disease, as it affects mankind in everyday life. It had, in fact, for many years been observed by competent observers that children who had mottled teeth had less dental decay than had those whose teeth were not mottled. This observation has been confirmed by so many serious investigators that it cannot be disclaimed. Being a factor of scientific value, it could not be ignored, and it led certain Public Health authorities to the assumption that at last the eternal problem of dental decay could be solved by nothing but the addition of fluorine to those water supplies which were deficient in it. As for the quantity of fluorine to be added to the drinking water, they knew well enough that the substance was a highly potent poison, not to be played with. To make the procedure appear safe, however, they discovered, as if by magic, that it was not a concentration of 1 p.p.m., but one of 1.5 p.p.m. that produced mottling of the teeth as the first visible sign of a systemic disease. To avoid the unsightly appearance of the teeth and any other concomitant signs of poisoning, it would, therefore, be quite within the limits of safety, they said, to make up a lower concentration, say, one of 1.2 p.p.m. to be ingested.

This kind of sophisticated reasoning had to be rejected outright for various reasons. In the first instance it is based on misrepresentation of facts, which were arrived at after most painstaking investigations carried out over a number of years by great scientists all over the world, particularly in this country. The findings obtained could not be allowed to be thrown overboard without valid scientific reason, simply to suit the occasion. The proposed concentration of 1.2 p.p.m. of fluorine was to be looked upon, therefore, as being in excess of that concentration which causes mottling of the teeth and other signs of chronic fluorine poisoning.

Furthermore, the reduced incidence of dental decay in children, who were ingesting small quantities of fluorine during the period of calcification of their permanent teeth, that is to say, from birth to the age of 8 years, is not lasting. Investigation has shown that, after the age of 8 years, the advantage of those children who were drinking water that contained fluorine over those who were not, was wiped out. The incidence of dental decay became equalized and, as the children grew older, it was as little influenced by their having ingested fluorine in their first 8 years of life as it was in those who have not ingested any at all. This fact leads, therefore, to the obvious conclusion that fluorine is not capable of preventing dental decay, as claimed by the advocates of adding fluorine to the drinking water, but only of delaying its onset.

Moreover, it is admitted on all sides that not all the children who were ingesting fluorine were free from dental decay whilst ingesting it. The percentage stated varies with the enthusiasm of the protagonists of adding fluorine to the drinking water. This procedure has now become known as "fluoridation", and its supporters as "fluoridators".

Worse still, to have their own way, many of the fluoridators were not acting in good faith, when they suppressed reports which were warnings against fluoridation of the drinking water as likely to do incalculable harm to the health of the population of this country, whilst in their widely publicized writings and discussions of the problem they brought out only those reports that suited their convenience.

In accepting the statement made by several reliable and trustworthy investigators to the effect that fluorine does, even if only temporarily, exert a beneficial influence on the onset of dental decay, I have in all fairness tried to explain this phenomenon by quoting a fundamental physiological law, according to which "if administered in a sufficiently reduced quantity, any poison will, in its sphere of influence, act no more in a deleterious but in a beneficial manner". This law applies as much to fluorine as it does to arsenic or any other poison which is used in Medicine under the strict supervision of the medical attendant.

Many years ago, a suggestion was in all seriousness made that to eradicate an epidemic of congenital syphilis prevalent at the time, small doses of arsenic should be added to the drinking water of every pregnant woman, because it is known that small doses of arsenic are beneficial in the treatment of syphilis. The suggestion was turned down by the medical profession as too ludicrous to be worthy of discussion.

The value of any idea, be it big or small, is, I believe, nowhere appreciated more than it is in this country. However insignificant it might initially appear to be, it may, and on occasion it does, lead to great developments in every field of human activity. If built on a foundation of strict honesty, it is sooner or later sure to be hailed as a great discovery which will ultimately benefit humanity. The first developments in the study of mottling of the teeth are amongst the latest achievements of the kind.

The idea of advocating fluorine for the prevention of dental decay is, however, not new. As many as 60 years ago a British investigator suggested that fluorine should be added to food, so as to reduce the incidence of dental caries. Fifteen years later a German recommended that, since lack of fluorine seemed to be an important factor in causing dental disease, fluorine should be given with a view to its prevention. Nothing more was heard of the idea either in Great Britain or in Germany, until it was recently revived in this country. Whereas, however, neither of the previous investigators went beyond recommending fluorides for prevention of dental decay, in this country an attempt has been and is still being made to force the ingestion of the poison by adding it to the public water supply.

An enlightened community will concede everybody the right to express and to promote his ideas, whatever their nature. It becomes, however, intolerable when these ideas are proffered to a public uninformed on the subject, in a manner which might convey that they are based on undisputed facts.

Chapter 21: Fluoridators At Work In U.S.A. And Elsewhere

Whilst the war was still on, I was in correspondence with the Dental Research Section of the Public Health Service, Bethesda, Maryland, who were in charge of the study of the subject of mottled teeth from every standpoint. They were familiar with my work on the medical aspect of chronic fluorine poisoning, of which mottled teeth are generally accepted as representing only one, an external visible sign, and they also knew of my intention to come and live in this country with a view to continuing my research work. It was natural, therefore, that on my arrival in this country I should pay them a courtesy visit, at which matters of mutual interest would be discussed. I realized by then that the project of adding fluorine to the public water supplies was launched and propagated from that centre. It was thus obvious that in our discussion a conflict of views would inevitably arise regarding the supposed beneficial effect of fluoridation on the teeth on the one hand and the grave harm done to the rest of the body on the other. Never-the-less, I earnestly hoped that an opportunity might be afforded to discuss whether a basis could be found on which the opposed points of view could be reconciled.

In the course of our discussion, I was informed that children living in an experimentally fluoridated area were examined for any harmful effects of the fluorine added to the public water supply, as compared with children who were living in an adjacent "control" area, to whose public water supply no fluorine had been added. I was greatly surprised when I was told that none of the various signs and symptoms of chronic fluorine poisoning, as reported in my published articles, were found in any of the children living in the fluoridated area. Not one! As if in an after-thought, however, it was quickly added: Oh, yes, "mottled nails", those little chalky-white or milk-white specks, patches and horizontal lines were in fact observed to occur much more frequently on the finger-nails of the children in the fluoridated than in the "control" area. I gave a sigh of relief. So they would not after all suggest that my findings were nothing but an outgrowth of my imagination! I contented myself with reminding them that I was the first to have drawn attention to this, the second, (and of the two probably even the more important because more easily detectable) external sign of the action of fluorine, which deprives the body of calcium via the parathyroid glands.

In our discussion, I enquired whether the children were examined in the same way as were the large number of recruits examined by me in the military camps during the war, as recorded in my papers which were published in medical journals. "No", was the reply, "the examination was not as systematic as yours was. We were guided by general impressions rather than by minute examination." I was happy to conclude that I was talking to a very honest man.

Of course, no signs and symptoms of chronic fluorine poisoning would be detected, if not looked for; and, of course, many of these would not yet present themselves at this early stage of the experiment, because they had had no time yet to develop in these children. Give them fluorine for a few more years, and they will you may be sure, show, apart from "mottled teeth" and "mottled nails", other ectodermal lesions as evidence of parathyroid deficiency, and brown patches of skin as evidence of a lowered function of the adrenal glands. They may in due course become victims of eczema and of obstinate constipation, excessive gas formation in the stomach and intestine, and of attacks of colicky pain in the abdomen. As the children grow older, they may develop every one of the other signs and symptoms of chronic tetany, which I had observed over a period of 25 years. They may later crowd the hospitals as chronic invalids, suffering from gastric and duodenal ulcers, from Bright's disease, from mental illness. And from cancer? No facilities are yet at hand to enable me to offer more than circumstantial evidence, which is not sufficient in a medical problem as grave as that of cancer.

In all fairness, accusations levelled at the Dental Research Section of the Public Health Service, Bethesda, Maryland, that their project of fluoridation is liable in the long run seriously to undermine the health of the nation do not appear to be fully justified. I have said enough in the previous chapters to emphasize the great debt of gratitude mankind owes American scientists, including those at Bethesda, for the discovery of facts which cannot fail to lead one day to further momentous discoveries. Unfortunately, the trouble seems to have arisen when some of the dental research workers, not content with their scientific achievements in the sphere of Dentistry, transgressed their field of competence and, without adequately consulting the medical profession, relied on their own judgment. The medical profession, in turn, continued to sit on the fence.

Recommendations based on fallacious premises were handed out to subordinate agencies, whose job it was to popularize the idea of fluoridation and to bring it into action. Two agencies were recruited for the purpose, namely, the Public Health Officers of the municipal councils, both medical and dental, and employees of the Water Works Organizations, all civil servants whose business it is to carry out instructions, however unpalatable they may be. Although cases are known in which Dental Public Health Officers and Water

Works Commissioners dared express their disagreement with the project of fluoridation, and successfully counselled its rejection by the City Councils, many of these civil servants propagated fluoridation effectively by employing methods which were no credit to advocates of a procedure purporting to eradicate dental decay in man. [1]At a conference, State Dental Directors and Public Health Officers were enlightened on how the population can, by gross misrepresentation of the facts, be won over in favor of fluoridation. In this process, they were told that, "the medical audience is the easiest audience in the world to present this to," as well as, "the Parent-Teacher Association (PTA) is a honey when it comes to fluoridation." Those in responsible position were warned, "If you can, I say if you can, because five times we have not been able to do it, keep fluoridation from going to a referendum."

As time went on, however, public opinion became better informed and often either voted by referendum against fluoridation or even stopped it after it had been in operation for some time. Outside help became necessary for the fluoridators, and the attempt to eradicate dental decay by means of the addition of the poison to the public water supplies had to be extended to foreign countries all over the world. Any successes obtained there, would be a welcome aid in winning over a vacillating public in this country. The same crude methods were employed abroad, through the agencies of Public Health Medical and Dental officers and Water Works Directors. If necessary, why, the good old, always dependable, "smear tactics", would be brought into the field of battle, as they had often enough proved reliable in this country, against all those who were honestly opposed to what they considered an objectionable tampering with the drinking water. The English and Scotch, Canadians, Australians, New Zealanders and Germans, all became a target for propaganda in favour of fluoridation. Agents could easily be found in most countries, willing to spread the gospel of the "beneficial" effect of fluorine on the teeth of mankind.

---

[1] Original text: At a conference, State Dental Directors and Public Health Officers were enlightened on how the population can by gross misrepresentation of the facts be won over in favor of fluoridation. In this process, "the medical audience is the easiest audience in the world to present this to", they were told, and "the Parent-Teacher Association (PTA) is a honey when it comes to fluoridation." "If you can, I say if you can, because five times we have not been able to do it, keep fluoridation from going to a referendum," those in responsible position were warned.

The "Chadwick Lecture" is delivered in London biennially on a subject bearing upon the improvement of public health. The lecturer is selected from amongst applicants who feel that they have something to contribute towards the advancement of medical knowledge for the benefit of mankind. On my release from the army, I applied for the honour of delivering the "Chadwick Lecture" on the subject of chronic fluorine poisoning, but my application was turned down. In 1952, however, the "Chadwick Lecture" was delivered on the action of fluorine by the Director of Water examination, Metropolitan Water Board, London, that colonel of the Royal Army Medical Corps with whom on my joining the army in 1941 I had the privilege of discussing the problem of the London drinking water over a cup of tea in the Officers' Mess of the Royal Army Medical College. The distinguished lecturer now appears to be better informed about the dental aspect of the action of fluorine than he was then, judging by the fact that he was now in a position to recite every one of the arguments adduced in favour of fluoridation of the drinking water in this country as applying also to the London drinking water. He is well acquainted with my work on chronic fluorine poisoning; yet, having now become an expert on the subject of fluorine, he brushed aside mine as well as any other opposition against fluoridation by saying that "such findings are at variance with the bulk of evidence," without even mentioning what those findings were. According to him, "further experiments (on fluorine) are unnecessary."

Since that discussion in the Officers' Mess of the Royal Army Medical College much water has flown under Westminster Bridge in London. On that occasion, the Director of Water Examination, Metropolitan Water Board, expressed his anxiety about frequent complaints that the London drinking water was the cause of a nasty taste in the mouth and of halitosis encountered amongst the population at large. I could not give him any information on this point then, but on looking out for this condition amongst those whom I examined for signs and symptoms of chronic fluorine poisoning, I found that his anxiety was fully justified.

An intelligent nation perseveres in demanding a reply to the following pertinent questions:

(1) Since all the statements made by the opponents of fluoridation can presumably be checked by responsible investigators, why is it that the fluoridators still adhere to their plans of adding fluorine to the public water supplies, before these statements are checked for their accuracy?

(2) Who is behind this attempt to ruthlessly exploit the health of the nation, nay, the health of humanity, with the help of unsuspecting, deficiently informed fluoridators?

(3) Is it the material gain expected to accrue to vested interests, which formerly had no alternative but to throw away the waste product of the fluorine-bearing cryolite that is unavoidably employed in the manufacture of aluminium, but which, following the discovery that small quantities of fluorine ingested during the first 8 years of life are capable of delaying by a few years (but by no means preventing) the onset of dental decay, are today trying to place them on the market for human consumption?

On a precise answer to these and similar questions depend the health and life of countless numbers of human beings all over the world.

Chapter 22: Otosclerosis: Gradually Increasing Deafness

In 1943 I had a paper published in a London medical journal on a condition in which gradually progressive deafness, leading to the victim ultimately becoming stone-deaf, is the principal feature. The cause has been looked for in vain ever since it was first described in the middle of the 18th century. A notable step towards its elucidation was made, however, not more than 35 years ago when it was found that this form of deafness was frequently associated with chronic tetany.

The fact that the deleterious effect of fluorine consists in its depriving the body of calcium has already been emphasized as being firmly established, and not likely ever to be disputed. Calcium is one of the indispensable materials deposited in the body, mainly in the bones, teeth, nails, etc. The milk-white or chalky-white markings seen on the teeth and nails in chronic fluorine poisoning are the result of decalcification of these tissues. It is likewise well-known that fluorine also inflicts severe damage on the skeleton. The bones become rarefied, porous and brittle, and break easily as a result of a slight accident. The tendons and ligaments become rigid and the surrounding soft tissues are deprived of their elasticity, causing stiffness which when affecting the spinal column produces a rounded back and impaired mobility of the trunk.

A further study of the slowly increasing deafness frequently occurring in association with chronic tetany suggested itself as a matter of urgency. It revealed that in this form of deafness, called otosclerosis, the bone in the skull, in which the inner ear apparatus is located, undergoes profound changes. It is studded with numerous milk-white or chalky-white patches of decalcification of variable sizes, which are identical with those observed in "mottled teeth" and "mottled nails" respectively. The deafness is often accompanied by ectodermal lesions and by patches of brown skin, amongst other signs of chronic fluorine poisoning. The nerves supplying the inner ear are also frequently affected, leading to severe attacks of dizziness and to noises in the ears which are sometimes said to be unbearable.

In connexion with all these findings, the fact that otosclerosis is frequently associated with chronic tetany which, as we now know, is caused by the long-continued action of fluorine on the parathyroid glands, led to the logical conclusion that there is no longer any need to look upon it as a mysterious condition, but that it may be classed amongst the other signs and symptoms of chronic fluorine poisoning. It would, however, be idle to assume that it can be improved by treatment directed against chronic fluorine poisoning. As in "mottled teeth", the damage to the bone housing the inner ear apparatus is permanent, but it is reasonable to expect that this treatment may prevent further deterioration. The only hope of eradicating the disease lies in its prevention, that is to say, in strictly avoiding fluorine, from whatever source it may come.

There are many people in London suffering from this form of deafness, but I was profoundly shocked when in the course of not more than a few days following my arrival in New York, I noticed in the streets and in other public places an uncommonly large number of people dependent on hearing aids. The question that immediately entered my mind was why it is that no one appears to have commented on this — to say the least — very unusual state of affairs. Surely, it must have struck other medical men before me; or am I to attribute any such omission to the fact that anything that is commonplace is not noticed by those who see it every day?

No doubt working medically in different countries under variable conditions stood me in good stead and gave me ample opportunity to compare things purely medical. Observing in this country certain signs and symptoms of disease, the co-existence of which would in ordinary circumstances appear baffling, did not present, therefore, the slightest difficulty in interpretation, since they were a replica of what I had observed in England for many years. They seem, however, to be more pronounced in this than in any other country. In spite of statistics to the contrary, invalidism appears to be rife, rising everywhere by leaps and bounds. The ascription of the rapidly growing incidence of "old" and the appearance of "new" diseases to superior medical knowledge and to improved technical diagnostic facilities is not acceptable. Hospitals for chronic diseases are crowded to capacity, and to make beds available for new arrivals invalids are sent to charitable institutions, where they will spend the remaining years of their life.

When I left London for the United States, my interest in the problem of "mottled teeth" seemed to be exhausted. What I needed to know about them I had learned from the study of the extensive literature on the subject and in the course of the several surveys which I had carried out in the British army. Henceforth, the knowledge acquired would serve me as a springboard for the continued study of co-existent signs and symptoms.

The question frequently asked was how fluorine could be blamed as a cause of so numerous diverse diseases. I believe that the evidence so far adduced gives a comprehensive picture of the mechanism involved in the action of fluorine. Being a nerve poison, fluorine affects the entire nervous system, its central, peripheral and vegetative sections. From the damage inflicted upon any one of them derive secondarily the various signs and symptoms of the many-sided disease.

Only when I arrived in this country did I become aware of the extent of the heated controversy over the proposed addition of fluorine to the public water supplies. A flood of correspondence reached me from every corner of this country and from some parts of Canada, requesting me to help in the matter. Being as yet a stranger, I could do no more than lend moral support to the opponents of the project. Soon, however, I found myself on the platform, addressing large public meetings which were organized for the purpose of fighting fluoridation in different parts of the country. Lantern slides, which I had prepared in the course of my research work, showed the audience the extent of damage produced by the ingestion of fluorine in man and in experimental animals. It caused the public bitter resentment to find out that up till now only the allegedly beneficial effect of fluorine on the teeth had been presented to them in support of fluoridation, but that the harmful effects on the remainder of the body were deliberately suppressed.

Even more significant was the fact that dentists, whom by invitation I was privileged to address at various meetings on the subject of chronic fluorine poisoning, found that they had been completely misinformed. They put the blame for it on their dental organizations, which in their professional journals gave them only one side of the picture of fluoridation.

I had already been warned against, and I soon became acquainted with, the smear tactics that would be directed against me personally and against my work by some sections of the fluoridators. Unable to refute my clinical observation on man and my experimental findings on animals, and irritated by the effectiveness of the lantern slides which faithfully depicted every stage of my work, they resorted to methods not worthy of those wishing to gain the confidence of the people. To those taken unawares these methods are distasteful, but I myself quickly became used to the sinister technique adopted. However foul, it had to be ignored. Lowering the standard to their level would inevitably result in inflicting damage on the cause itself. A quarrel picked on a side issue by hecklers at public meetings may quite well have been the aim of the fluoridators in their endeavour to get the discussion off the straight line of debate, so as to discredit the arguments adduced against their plans. I have so far not been accused of subversive actions in connexion with my work on the subject of fluorine!

Whatever fate might have in store for me, the addition of fluorine to the drinking water and forcing the population at large, irrespective of the fact that it had no influence on their teeth after the age of 8 years, thereby increasing the amount of the poison already ingested with numerous articles of food and drink to a level which is bound in the long run to cause illness, had from the purely medical point of view to be fought through thick and thin. As I saw it, for a medical man familiar with the grave risk involved, to sit back with folded arms would be tantamount to an act of dishonesty and betrayal of the trust and implicit confidence reposed in him by suffering humanity.

Fluoridation has proved to be a powerful obstacle in my long struggle against chronic fluorine poisoning. Not only would patients already suffering from this be doomed to greater suffering because of the larger amounts of the poison which they were now required to swallow with their drinking water, but all those less susceptible, who had hitherto succeeded in escaping the ravaging effect of fluorine, would be subjected to an increased dosage. In short, in place of having its health improved by the cutting off of every source of fluorine intake, this nation is invited to submit to gradual self-destruction by ingesting more of the rat poison. This certainly seems wrong to any logically thinking person.

My own attempt to deliver humanity of its Public Enemy Number One will continue. In conjunction with the work of all those others opposed to fluoridation of the public water supplies it cannot fail to bear fruit eventually.

Chapter 23: Old Soldiers Never Die

I did not leave England, where I spent 30 years of my life, with a light heart or for trivial reasons. It was for not less a purpose than to try to bring the results of my work on chronic fluorine poisoning to a level at which I hope they would benefit suffering humanity. My desire was to obtain facilities in this country in hospitals for chronic diseases, where I could utilize my findings for alleviating, if not for curing, some of those chronic illnesses which I believed could fairly be ascribed to the long-continued ingestion of toxic amounts of fluorine.

I mentioned my plans during my visit to the Dental Research Section of the United States Public Health Service, Bethesda, but was informed that I could expect no assistance from that quarter, although if it were my desire to submit an application for a grant to carry on my work, forms would be furnished upon request. In fact, a few days later I received a neatly packed collection of forms, weighing not less than three quarters of a pound, and containing Instructions, 27 of them with 15 subsections explaining how to apply for a grant, and a Statement of Policy of the Division of Research Grants, National Institute of Health, Bethesda, embodying 13 sections with 34 paragraphs. To supply additional information necessary for objective evaluation, the applicant is required to provide 40 copies of supplemental material in manuscript form, on top of the application forms duly filled in. Never having had any experience of the financial aspect of my work I felt that the matter contained in the application forms could be better handled by a chartered accountant or a capable business manager than by myself, unless it could be done by the official of an institution in which the work was to be carried out.

To find such an institution would be the hardest part of my task. My experience gained in London after my release from the British army, and before I succeeded in obtaining facilities to carry out animal experiments at the Department of Physiology, Middlesex Hospital Medical School, was enough to make me fight shy of a repetition of the struggle. Being a stranger in this country, and being known through my writings mainly to those whose ideas on fluorine were diametrically opposed to my own, I could not expect to surmount this difficulty. If I approached any of the hospitals for facilities to carry out the proposed work, I should have to lay my request before that very authority which proposed the addition of fluorine to the drinking water. Any such approach to an institution whose decision would depend on the Public Health Service would, therefore, be time wasted.

I wrote to the American Cancer Society, asking for facilities to carry out treatment directed against chronic fluorine poisoning on selected cases of inoperable cancer under the fullest supervision of the chief of any assigned hospital, or of his deputies. I gave an outline of that treatment and pointed out that the patients so treated would be completely unaware of any change in their mode of life. Apart from the preparation of the special diet in the kitchen, no additional personnel would be required to look after the patients, who would be segregated in a special ward. My letter did not contain a single word concerning a request for a grant.

The following was the reply from the Medical and Scientific Director of the American Cancer Society:

"The American Cancer Society does not own nor operate any facilities for conducting research, either fundamental or basic, and therefore I do not quite see how I can be helpful in opening up facilities in which you might carry forward your proposed studies. The Society does support research on a broad scale and in the case of research or the project type, into which class your proposal falls, the selection of recipients from among the numerous requests for grants-in-aid, is made by the Committee on Growth of the National Research Council. The Secretary of the Committee on Growth, whose address is 2101 Constitution Avenue, Washington 25, D. C., will provide you with more detailed information as to applications for grant-in-aid funds."

I immediately wrote a letter, similar to the previous one, to the Committee on Growth, National Research Council, Washington, D. c., and received the following reply:

"In reply to your letter of 10 November 1952, I am enclosing application blanks to be used in applying for a grant in cancer research, a brochure which describes these grants, a booklet explaining policies and procedures, and a special form on which the investigator is requested to summarize briefly the work he proposes to do. This form should be filled out and returned with the application.

"I hasten to add that I am sending this material to you only so you can see the type of program which the Committee on Growth is carrying on. I regret very much that it does not appear the Committee on Growth can be of any assistance to you, at least not in the immediate future. From the enclosed material you will note that applications for grants must be received prior to 1 October to be considered during the winter. Grants recommended during the winter become effective on the following 1 July. Under these circumstances applications received during the coming months cannot be considered until a year from this time and grants recommended at that time will not become effective until 1 July 1954.

"You also will note from the enclosed material that grants are awarded only to institutions and not to individuals. Therefore, it will be necessary for you to arrange an affiliation with a reputable university, hospital or research institution before your application could be considered.

"In regard to the possibility of making laboratory and necessary facilities available to you, I also am afraid that the Committee can be of no assistance. Neither the Committee nor the National Research Council has any laboratories of their own nor do they support specific laboratories financially. Therefore, the Committee has no facilities which could be assigned to you. In the past, the Committee has consistently refused to take the responsibility of requesting independent institutions to make facilities available to a particular investigator and I am sure this policy will be maintained in the future.

"I am sorry indeed that it appears simply impossible for the Committee on Growth to be of any help to you at the moment. However, if any questions arise on which you think I might have some information, please do not hesitate to let me know."

No questions arose, however, on which I required further information. The position was perfectly clear! My approach to the problem through the regular channels would lead me nowhere. It is no use trying to break down the barriers of red tape, whether in this country or in England. There is something radically wrong where medical research is concerned. I very much doubt whether any business concern, be it large or small, would be able to carry on its activities for any length of time by using methods similar to those used by the highest medical institutions in this country, designed to promote research for the benefit of humanity. I often wondered whether these institutions, supported as they are by vast sums of money, both public and private, would not do much better by appointing a panel of capable business men to organize and administer matters for them.

Hoping against hope, I approached the Memorial Center for Cancer and Allied Diseases and received the following reply:

"I read your letter and your paper "Pathological Findings in Fluorine Intoxication" with very great interest. However, I should like to point out that this is out of the area of our interest and would suggest that you refer it to United States Public Health Service." And a fortnight later: "Thank you for sending your curriculum vitae. I find that you have done some very interesting work. I do wish that

117

our space were not so terribly limited so that we could accommodate additional workers on our research staff. However, this is the present condition and we are unable to offer you anything here."

The favourable outcome, recorded in a previous chapter of the treatment directed against chronic fluorine poisoning in one patient, and the partial improvement in another at a mental hospital in London, suggested the necessity of further research on a larger number of patients suffering from mental illness. I wrote a letter to this effect to the State Commissioner of Mental Hygiene, Albany, N. Y. The following was the reply:

"This is in response to your letter of October 18, 1952, concerning fluoride detoxication in the treatment of mental disorder. "I regret to say that the Department of Mental Hygiene is not in a position to take direct action on such matters, since this is a procedure to be passed by the Director of each institution. His decision as to the project would necessarily depend upon the availability of personnel and other local factors."

At hospitals for chronic diseases, every endeavour to get permission to carry out the proposed work came to nothing because of my age. When I started my investigation on the subject of fluorine at the age of 38 years, and also during the years that followed, I was too young to be listened to. Having in the course of the years obtained important results from my work I am now pronounced to be too old, and prevented from carrying them into effect by the hospitals' regulations, which decree that at the age of 65 years no medical man shall continue to work within the walls of any hospital. So the old adage is true which says that the age of a medical man is never right; he is either too young or he is too old. It follows that, if red tape has its own way, I am at the age of 65 years to be prevented from carrying on my life-long work to a final conclusion. The veil of mystery surrounding certain diseases of a hitherto obscure origin is not to be allowed to be lifted, now or at any time, and the ravaging effect of ingesting toxic amounts of fluorine is to continue unabated. During the war, a Tommy in the British army brought me an amusing little quatrain, which he found in a humorous magazine. It read:

"Of old when folk lay sick and sorely tried,
The doctors gave them physic, and they died.
But here's a happier age; for now we know,
both how to make men sick and keep them so."

It is, of course, not true to suggest that doctors make men sick. At any rate, at the time this clever little poem was written, there was as yet no question of adding to the public water supplies fluorine to make men sick. When the question did arise, medical men were not consulted. It is, however, time to say that those amongst them who believe that certain illnesses could be prevented and alleviated are not permitted to share their knowledge with the medical profession at large.

A dreaded "new" disease, which made its appearance not more than some 30 years ago, is cancer of the lung. Search is going on all over the world, but its cause continues to resist every effort at its elucidation. There is not the slightest doubt that its incidence is rapidly increasing everywhere.

It occurred to me that, since the long-continued ingestion of toxic amounts of fluorine is believed to be capable through its action on the vegetative nervous system of producing cancer in different parts of the body, including the lungs, any fluorine found to be present in tobacco might act as superadded local irritant in the production of cancer of the lung.

In 1948 I had a paper published in a leading medical journal in Sweden in which I recorded the presence of fluorine in the tobacco smoke obtained from a lighted cigarette. In 1950 while discussing the problem of inoperable cancer with Professor R.W. Scarff, Director of the Bland-Sutton Institute of Pathology at the Middlesex Hospital and Secretary of the British Empire Cancer Campaign, I drew his attention to this important finding and its possible bearing on the cause of lung cancer, as well as to the possible role of fluorine in general in the causation of cancer in any part of the body. A committee investigating the role which smoking might play in the causation of cancer of lung had sent out a circular in 1951 to every medical man in Great Britain to inquire about their smoking habits, and to invite observations made on themselves and on their patients with reference to the effect of smoking on their respiratory tract. In my reply, I suggested the advisability of following up my findings recorded in the Swedish medical journal.

I do not know whether the British Empire Cancer Campaign or the committee investigating the possible relationship of smoking and cancer of the lung has ever taken note of the presence of fluorine in tobacco, as recorded by me for the first time. Nor have I had, so far, access to the official report on the 30th annual general meeting of the former, held recently in London. I am reliably informed, however, that in his report on progress in the field of cancer research, Professor A. Haddow, Director of the Chester Beatty Research Institute of the Royal Cancer Hospital, had said:

"We have accumulated knowledge of sore hundreds of pure chemical agents, of different types but all endowed with a remarkable capacity to induce cancer. In the case of certain cancer cells, we have now recognized, for the first time, the imprint left upon them by the chemical agents which induced their appearance."

Later in his speech, Professor Haddow said:

"Whilst much remains to be done, I would hazard the prediction that sooner or later, depending on our efforts, we shall see in the chemotherapy of cancer something entirely new, namely, a kind of substitution therapy by which the cancer cell will be controlled from without. Even cancer prevention, which only a few years ago seemed utterly beyond our hopes, may yet prove to be within our ultimate powers. The possibility is suggested that coal smoke and tobacco smoking may act together after the manner of a carcinogen (cancer-producing substance) and a co-carcinogen."

It is refreshing to see from this report that the investigation into the origin of cancer appears now to be centered on chemical agents damaging normal cells, thereby turning them into cancer cells. It has not yet been remarked that fluorine is one of those cancer-producing chemical agents, but it is perhaps not far-fetched to assume that the substance which may need substituting is that calcium which has been taken away by the long-continued action of fluorine. If this is so, nothing except denying facilities to carry out treatment directed against chronic fluorine poisoning can stop us from curing and, in due course, from preventing cancer

As for cancer of the lungs, it is well-known that coal smoke contains fluorine. The sum total of fluorine derived from coal, from tobacco and from the numerous articles of food and drink in everyday life is sufficient to be regarded as the long-sought cause of the greatest scourge of the human race.

In this country a group has recently been appointed under the direction of Dr. Paul Kotin, Department of Pathology, University of Southern California, School of Medicine, Los Angeles, to investigate any relationship between air pollution and cancer of the lungs. I have drawn the attention of Dr. Kotin to the fact that I detected fluorine in tobacco smoke and received the following reply:

"Thank you for your interest in our project. Should the expansion of our studies require an evaluation of fluorine as an air pollutant you may be sure I will refer to your work and to you personally."

Chapter 24: Postscript

Having come to the end of my story, I should very much like in all humility to assure those who believe that every effort at penetrating the darkness of Nature is merely waste of time that the results of the work here recounted have not come to me as a gift from heaven. It required some 30 years of incessant toil, for which not the slightest financial reward was forthcoming. On the contrary, I myself had to bear out of my own pocket the cost of several laboratory examinations. All I am now concerned with is that the attention of the general public may widely be drawn to the issues involved, for they bear upon the health of the public themselves.

The problem of fluorine is not a new one by any means. Like other elements in nature, the known ones and those as yet unknown, fluorine was there all the time as an important constituent of the earth's crust. It always played its part in inflicting grave harm on mankind, but it invariably succeeded in resisting every attempt at being brought to light as an important cause of human suffering. It was not until the momentous discovery was made by American science that "mottled teeth" were produced by the long-continued ingestion of small amounts of fluorine that its significance became known to the dental profession and thence to the general public.

There can be little doubt that, in spite of all the work done on the subject, things would have continued unchanged, as in most cases they do in medical matters, and that the deleterious effect not only on the teeth but on every other organ in the human body would have been left uninvestigated indefinitely were it not for a small group of American dentists who originally proposed the addition of fluorine to the public water supplies. Paradoxically, this fact will one day be hailed as an important milestone in inspiring medical research and in helping to achieve practical results towards alleviating human suffering. It stimulated, more powerfully than anything else would have done, the interest in the problem of fluorine amongst the population at large. The subject became a popular theme of discussion everywhere, particularly since it was looked upon not as something belonging to the dead past, but as a problem of urgent present interest.

It is fair to say that it was because of the absence of guidance on the part of those who were normally looked upon as the guardians of the nation's health that for the first time in the history of Medicine people in various parts of the country began to try to take the matter concerning their health and the health of future generations into their own hands. They realized that the medical profession, preoccupied with its endeavour to help its patients according to prevailing standards, had no leisure to take part in the discussion of a problem as controversial as was that of fluorine. More important still, people made up their minds that those few amongst the medical profession who did take any interest in the problem and did condemn the addition of fluorine to the public water supplies as an evil action were as helpless as they were themselves with regard to official medical policy and were unable to exert any influence on its course. Indeed, some amongst those few thought it more expedient to withhold their opinion, since it might embroil them in a dispute with their professional organizations and with some of their patients.

The general public began to be alarmed at the prospect of eventually becoming victims of chronic disease through the long-continued ingestion of toxic amounts of fluorine forced upon them and at the thought that, even without the addition of fluorine to the drinking water, certain signs and symptoms of an obscure illness amongst themselves and amongst their relatives and friends might be nothing but unrecognized effects of chronic fluorine poisoning, resulting from the ingestion of quantities of the poison that contaminated numerous articles of their daily food and drink. They insisted that the authorities responsible for the health of the nation should defer any action in the matter of fluoridation until it was proved beyond the slightest shadow of doubt that the ingestion of any further quantities of fluorine added to the drinking water would involve no increased risk for the population. They deplored and rejected all statements of misinformed or unscrupulous professional propagandists to the effect that fluorine was good for them.

It was obvious that the vast majority of members of the medical profession had never even heard of the large amount of literature that was published on the subject, and the public urged their medical advisers to become informed on the problem of fluorine. The demand was particularly strong where the patients appeared to be better acquainted with the subject than were their medical advisers, whose attention had to be drawn to the existence of a large number of publications dealing with complaints, seemingly identical with those of the patients, that were caused by the ingestion of fluorine. I had requests coming from people living in different parts of the country asking for a list of my own publications, which they wished to pass on to their medical advisers for study. Whilst the manuscript of "The Drama of Fluorine" was being prepared it was suggested that this list should be incorporated for the benefit of all those who might be interested.

Public opinion insists that the study of the problem of fluorine shall embrace not only its dental aspect but also the general effect of the poison on the whole body. Many pleaded that the work which I had carried out in England should be verified in all its details, and that it should be ascertained whether the findings obtained there applied with equal force in this country. They are confident that common sense will prevail in the end concerning the wanton addition to the public water supplies of a poison as potent as fluorine. Not content, however, with the slow progress so far achieved in the fight against certain diseases of mankind, they hope that the effort aiming at the elucidation and eventual elimination of those diseases will be extended in any direction that may prove promising. They expect that the utmost endeavour shall be made to investigate whether such diseases as recurrent gastric and duodenal ulcers, Bright's disease and cancer in any part of the body can be favourably influenced by treatment directed against chronic fluorine poisoning and that separate wards will be reserved for this purpose in specially assigned hospitals for chronic diseases. They ardently hope that the project will not founder on cook's threat to give notice to leave because of the additional work in the hospital's kitchen.

The same applies to the urgent necessity to take appropriate steps towards answering the question whether this treatment will succeed in doing for large numbers of inmates of mental hospitals in this country what it did in two cases at a hospital on the outskirts of London. I cannot believe that in the United States of America the lack of nurses, however acute it may generally be, will stand in the way of trying to find out whether this method of treatment in cases of mental disease accompanied by patches of brown pigmentation of the skin, the first ever to be attempted in the history of psychiatry, will succeed in doing more for these poor victims than the methods hitherto applied have done.

As for nerve-leprosy which has been discussed in a previous chapter, it must be realized that no treatment can be expected to undo structural damage to the peripheral nervous system and all its consequences. It would, however, be of the greatest value for the study of this disease to survey a large number of patients at a leprosarium with a view to ascertaining whether there is a statistically significant proportion amongst them who exhibit co-existent signs and symptoms of chronic fluorine poisoning,

*   *   *

Nearly two years have passed since I arrived in this country, hoping that facilities would be available to enable me to translate the results of my work hitherto obtained into practical action for the benefit of mankind. Even though, as described in the pages of this book, I have so far failed in arousing interest in the problem of chronic fluorine poisoning amongst those whose primary duty it should have been to study it without bias and prejudice, I take comfort in the belief that my modest contribution to the work on the subject of fluorine will, in the not too distant future, help to lighten the lot of suffering humanity.

§   §   §   §

AUTHOR'S LIST OF PUBLICATIONS IN MEDICAL JOURNALS

1. "Some Skin Manifestations and Their Relation to the Disturbance of the Gastro-Intestinal Tract." Franco-Brit. Med. Rev. 1928, 5, 1. Reprinted in American Medicine, 1928, n.s. 23, 913.

2. "Chronic Poisoning by an Irritant Contained in Aluminium Cooking Utensils and Tap Water." Franco-Brit. Med. Rev. 1928 5, 61. Reprinted in American Medicine, 1929, n. s. 24, 40.

3. "The Clinical Aspect of Chronic Poisoning by Aluminium and Its Alloys." London, 1933.

4. "Fluorine." Lancet, 1941, 2, 23.

5. "Incidence of Mottled Teeth." Lancet, 1942, 1, 649.

6. "Mottled Teeth in Great Britain." Brit. Den. J. 1942, 73, 149.

7. "Classification of the Degree of Severity of Mottling of Teeth." Brit. Dent. J. 1942, 73, 233.

8. "Chronic Fluorine Poisoning (Fluorosis): Signs and Symptoms." Edinb. Med. J. 1942, 49, 707.

9. "Endemic Fluorosis in Great Britain." Edinb. Med. J. 1943, 50, 237.

10. "Fluorosis and the Parathyroid Glands." J. Hyg., Camb. 1942 42, 500.

11. "Mottled Nails: An Early Sign of Fluorosis." J. Hyg., Camb. 1943, 43, 69.

12. "Fluorine in Drinking Water." J. Hyg., Camb. 1943, 43, 142.

13. "Some Epithelial Changes in Fluorosis." J. Hyg., Camb. 1944, 43, 400. 1

14. "Incidence of Dystrophies in Organs Regulated by the Parathyroid Glands." J. Hyg., Camb. 1944, 43, 402.

15. "Fluorine Alopecia." J. Hyg., Camb. 1946, 44, 276.

16. "Some Skin Manifestations in Hypoparathyroidism." J. Hyg., Camb. 1947, 45, 93.

17. "The Aetiology of Otosclerosis." J. Laryngol. Otol. 1943, 58, 151.

18. "Disturbance of Pigmentation in Fluorosis." Acta Med. Scand., Stockholm, 1946, 126, 65. 141

19. "Congenital Ectodermal Dysplasia." Acta Med. Scand., Stockholm, 1947, 127, 570.

20. "Some Sources of Intake and Methods of Elimination of Fluorine." Acta Med. Scand., Stockholm, 1948, 130, 78.

21. "Disturbance of Pigmentation in a Half-Caste. Riehl's Melanosis. Poikiloderma of Civatte." Acta Derm. Venereol Scand., Stockholm, 1946, 27, 83.

22. "Riehl's Melanosis." Acta Derm. - Venereol. Scand., Stockholm 1949, 29, Z7. 23. "Varicose Veins and Fluorosis." Med. Press, 1948, 219, 106.

24. "Some Dermatoses in Fluorosis." Urol. Cutan. Rev. 1948, 52, 475.

25. "Stigmata of Degeneration in Fluorosis." Urol. Cutan. Rev., 1949, 53, 34.

26. "Experimental Fluorosis in Rats." Exp. Med. Surg. 1949, 7, 134.

27. "Fluorine and Vitamin B." Exp. Med. Surg. 1950, 8, 361.

28. "Pathological Findings in Fluorine Intoxication." Exp. Med. Surg. 1952, 10, 54.

29. "Further Study of the Role Played by Fluorine in the Causation of Disease." Exp. Med. Surg. 1952, 10, 63.

30. "Maculo-anaesthetic Leprosy and Fluorosis." Exp. Med. Sure;. 1952, 10 , 194.

31. "Riehl's Melanosis and the Adrenal Glands." Arch. Int. Med. 1950, 86, 682.

32. "Tetanoide Erscheinungen bei Chronischer Fluorveriftung." Deutsche Med. Wschr. 1951, 76, 1558.

33. "Riehl's Melanose." Schweiz. Med. Wschr. 1952, 82, 359.

34. "Therapie und Prophylaxe der Fluorschadigung." Ther. Gegenw. 1953, 92, 165.

Editor's Addendum

Nearly 70 years after this was originally published, we are still being poisoned by fluoride, most prevalent by fluoridation of our drinking water. Unfortunately, Dr Spira's work was not enough to stop the authorities from adding this poison to our drinking waters.

When the editor dedicated himself to losing weight by exercising and drinking copious quantities of water, his health diminished greatly. The municipal water he drank was fluoridated to 1.2 ppm. This led to learning about iodine deficiency and fluoride's role in it. Iodine is a nutrient and fluoride a poison. Fluoride interferes with iodine's biological function, uptake, and elimination. Because of this, the editor suffered many symptoms described in this book.

The editor recommends using fluoride-free water — either spring water or water filtered by reverse osmosis. These filtration systems are readily available.

The editor hopes that government authorities put an end to fluoridation of all types. It will take continued work to make the government act responsibly.

In the news are other types of fluoride pollution; one of them is known as C8. It has led to large lawsuits against the companies that made this pollution.

[Perfluorooctanoic acid, commonly known as PFOA or C8, is a "perfluorinated" chemical, which means that its base includes carbon chains attached to fluorine atoms.]

Additional Reading and Resources by Editor

- *The Fluoride Deception,* Christopher Bryson 2006 [Looks into the history and looks into answering the "Why?" of flouridation]
- *The Devil's Poison: How Fluoride Is Killing You,* Dean Murphy DDS 2008 [Review of the science biology and history]
- *Superman's Not Coming: Our National Water Crisis and What We the People Can Do About It,* Erin Brockovich 2020 [The battle]
- *The Iodine Crisis: What You Don't Know About Iodine Can Wreck Your Life,* Lynne Farrow and David Brownstein 2013 [Part of the cure.]
- *Iodine: Why You Need It, Why You Can't Live Without It,* M.D. David Brownstein 2014
- *Fluoride in Drinking Water: A Scientific Review of EPA's Standards.* National Research Council. 2006. The National Academies Press, Washington, DC: https://doi.org/10.17226/11571. [A government review of the literature.]
- *How My Eyes Were Healed Naturally And Yours Can Too: It's Not Because You're Over Forty,* Steve Fonseca 2017 [Part of the editor's story]
- *The Cure Of Imperfect Sight by Treatment Without Glasses*: Dr. Bates Original, First Book - *Natural Vision Improvement,* William H. Bates, Ophthalmologist William Horatio Bates M.D. 1920 [This book is available in many editions; try to find one that is an accurate copy]
- The Fluoride Action Network http://fluoridealert.org/(FAN) seeks to broaden awareness among citizens, scientists, and policymakers on the toxicity of fluoride compounds. FAN provides comprehensive and up-to-date information and remains vigilant in monitoring government agency actions that impact the public's exposure to fluoride

The Fluoride Action Network is currently suing the EPA for not fulfilling its responsibility. http://fluoridealert.org/issues/tsca-fluoride-trial/

Update on the ongoing TSCA Trial (As of August 2022)

Under the Toxic Substances Control Act (TSCA), a group of non-profits and individuals petitioned the U.S. Environmental Protection Agency in 2016 to end the addition of fluoridation chemicals into drinking water due to fluoride's neurotoxicity. The EPA rejected the petition. In response, the groups sued the EPA in Federal Court. The trial was held in June 2020 and, as of June 2022, the judge has yet to make his ruling.

Glossary

Aetiological:	Causing or contributing to the development of a disease or condition.
Ectodermal Lesions:	Skin Lesions: Acne, Boils, Nodules, Rash, Hives (Weals) etc.
Fluoride, Fluorine:	These terms in nearly all medical and news articles are interchangeable. In the field of chemistry there is a clear distinction, but it does not apply to normal usage.
Fluoridation:	The practise of adding fluoride to municipal water supposedly to lower the rate of dental caries (cavities). This is done in most municipalities in the USA. It results in the most significant exposure to Fluoride in the population.
Foetus:	Fetus
Fur:	Mineral and rust deposits in pipes.
Otosclerosis:	Is a condition in which there is abnormal bone growth inside the ear. Symptoms may include hearing loss or ringing in the ears. In rare cases, vertigo may occur.
Penulous:	Pendulous, hanging down.
Physic:	1) The art or practice of healing disease. 2) The practice or profession of medicine 3) A medicinal agent or preparation
Tetany:	A condition marked by intermittent muscular spasms, caused by malfunction of the parathyroid glands and a consequent deficiency of calcium.
Weals:	Wheals, hives